HOSPITALS, DOCTORS, PATIENTS

HOSPITALS, DOCTORS, PATIENTS

MEMORIES FROM
A COTTAGE INDUSTRY

Simeon Locke

To order additional copies of this book, contact:
Xlibris Corporation
1-888-795-4274
www.Xlibris.com
Orders@Xlibris.com
89421

CONTENTS

Je me souviens
Des jours anciens
Et je pleure

Verlaine

PREFACE

I opened the door to the waiting room to greet a new patient. An elderly man struggled to his feet and shuffled toward the office with bent knees, bent hips, bent arms and tremulous fingers. He clearly had Parkinsons disease. After the initial amenities I asked why he had come to see me. "I went to see my doctor," he said. "I didn't even get into his office when he said 'You've got Parkinsons disease.' How did he know? He didn't examine me. I need an expert."

I knew at once. He didn't need an expert; he needed time. He didn't need a diagnosis; that was evident. He didn't only need the course of medication that could be found in the books. He needed a relationship. He needed someone to listen, to explain, to understand, to explain again and to be available. He needed a doctor—the old-fashioned kind.

They are hard to find. The system discourages them. Training redirects them. The cost of health care goes up, the quality of care goes down. Technology improves, diagnosis is more accurate, treatment is more sophisticated but the quality of care declines. Francis W. Peabody pointed out that "the secret of the care of the patient is in caring for the patient". That is no longer possible. What had early in my life been a ministry—a compassionate calling as my father practiced it—became a scientific profession which then turned into its current form—a business. This was the natural result of what has been termed the monetization of medicine, an outgrowth of Medicare but also a reflection of what has occurred in all areas of society. Materialism, consumerism, and the emphasis on money have changed the patient into a consumer and the physician into a provider. As if the doctor were selling a commodity. Only John Falstaff could do that (Henry IV Part 2 II ii). "A good wit will make use of any thing: I will turn disease to commodity." Health cannot be bought and sold. The doctor does not provide health; at best what is provided is time. Time to use as the patient—the so-called consumer—chooses, for the patient is the major participant in the relationship. The doctor offers advice, guidance, suggestions; the patient evaluates and makes decisions. The decisions may be ill informed or destructive but they are the patients to make. Because a treatment program is right (that is, scientifically valid) does not mean it is best. What's best for a given patient depends on many things other than medical—beliefs, desires, attitudes, outlooks. The good doctor, the compassionate doctor gives opinions but remains non-judgemental and supportive even if the patient's choice of behavior is contrary to the doctor's suggestions.

Just as the patient needs time, so the doctor needs time and the system precludes that. The obscene notion that time is money—which I first encountered over fifty years ago on a sign (in English) on a functionary's desk in Paris—is implemented by the Insurance Carriers. Administrative nurses patrol the corridors and rap on the door when the time spent with a new patient exceeds fifteen minutes. As I said to the colleague who told us about that one day at lunch, if I had only fifteen minutes with each new patient I would certainly make mistakes, miss things and might be guilty of malpractice. "The HMO believes" he replied, "that if you are not sued for malpractice at least twice a year you are spending too much time with your patients". Fifteen minutes for a Chief Complaint, History of Present Illness, Past History, Family History, Social History, Review of Systems, Physical Examination, Diagnosis, Treatment Plan, and a dictated report, never mind a discussion with the patient. Another colleague accompanied his wife to her first visit to a Health Maintenance Organization. The doctor heard the current problem and examined her. My colleague asked, "Do we no longer take a Past History?" "We do that on the second visit" was the reply, signifying that time was short. And time is money.

What have got to change if the current system is to prevail are the patient's expectations. And with enough exposure, they will. But although what to expect from your doctor will adapt to what you receive time and time again, the need,—the emotional component of the "whole person" the doctor is taught to care for—will not. And so a neighbor I met at the Post Office told me that after seventeen years as a patient at a famous specialty clinic he found a new doctor closer to home who is "great because she listens." Previously he said he felt as if he were intruding in the relationship between his doctor and the doctor's computer.

Perhaps accuracy of diagnosis and appropriate treatment are enough. Perhaps the other needs are simply self-indulgence. But if, as a physician, you want to do the best you can for accuracy of diagnosis you need a relationship on which to build, to get information, to learn about your patient. As a young recruit in Navy Boot camp, I felt sick and reported to sick call. The newly minted doctor asked me "What's your chief complaint?" I did not know Chief Complaint was a technical term used to summarize symptoms. All I knew was that I was not there to complain; I was sick. I was offended he thought I was a complainer. So, I wasn't going to help him. When he saw the petechiae on my wrists (a sign of meningococcal meningitis) he said "You've got the measles" He had alienated me so I did not tell him I had already had the measles as a child, and I knew you didn't get the measles twice. Fortunately, at the Base Hospital to which he sent me, a second young doctor enlisted my participation, made the correct diagnosis, treated me with the newly manufactured sulfa drug, and cured me. The patient is a participant and must participate. Perhaps a machine can make the diagnosis but care of the patient cannot (and should not) be mechanical.

Many years ago, I was one of a three-member committee to consider the use by our hospital of computer-aided diagnosis. We visited a major medical center that was using computer-aided diagnosis so we could assess the utility and suitability for our hospital. The department was run be a hyperactive physician with what is called a Type A personality—the sort of man prone to develop gastric ulcer disease. We interacted with the computer and were impressed with the results. Having presented it with an initial symptom it asked a small number of questions then arrived at the correct diagnosis—the one we had decided in advance. I expressed my approval and said it was an impressive device. "Yes" said one of my committee colleagues," but I'll bet it never noticed the little bit of Maalox in the corner of its boss' mouth."

The medical community is more than just doctors and patients. Hospitals are a third part of it. Like the Federal Government, the medical community has three branches and like the Federal Government, the interaction among the three branches creates a dynamic tension and a resulting balance of power. That balance is not fixed; from time to time it shifts. For a long time—the era when it was believed that "knowledge is power"—the doctors were in charge for they had the knowledge. With deconstructionism and the various revolutions of the past decades, it was decided that power is bad so, according to the evident syllogism, knowledge is bad. The balance began to shift, aided by the contemporaneous increase of health insurance, including Medicare, with more power, more medical decision making shifted to the hospital. Simultaneously social attitudes—feminism among others—began to alter the relationship between doctor and patient. Paternalism was denigrated. The doctor was considered an adversary. The therapeutic relationship began to break down. Certain assumptions and implicit suppositions could no longer be relied on. If my patient felt he could not trust me, should I feel I could not trust my patient? At one time I had argued that when a used car salesman came into my office I believed everything he told me; when I went into his office I didn't believe a thing he said. The context of the interaction implied certain unspoken rules. As a doctor, I was on his side; as a salesman, he was an adversary. If my patient was now an adversary could I really be of help?

And what of the hospital? Here, too, in the decades following the 60's the relationship with doctors became increasingly adversarial. But the adversity was complicated—a love-hate relationship. It was the doctors after all who admitted patients—the source of revenue—to hospitals. And it was the hospital that provided services to the doctors and ultimately to their patients. But what had once been a cooperative venture increasingly became a tug of war. I remember, as an example, a medical staff meeting at which members elaborated a number of complaints about the hospital operated telephone answering service: messages were lost, not delivered, incorrect and patients were given faulty information. Instead of accepting the complaints as accurate and looking into them, trying to correct them, saying it would help, the Hospital administration stonewalled, denied the claims, said the doctors were wrong, the allegations were groundless. What should have been a joint problem, the solution of which would have been beneficial to both participants ended up unsolved and one more source of animosity between what should have been a pair of partners.

We talk of institutions or groups—hospitals, doctors, and patients—as if they were entities. They are of course actually aggregates of individuals—individuals who vary in personality, desire, needs, attitudes. And yet the groups or institutions develop personalities of their own, perhaps as a manifestation of the views of the dominant leaders, perhaps as a manifestation of group attitudes and behaviors within which individual attitudes and behaviors differ. The evolution of attitudes of the individuals to those of the group, then to the institution is reflected in the transition from ministry to profession to business. Individual morality becomes formalized by professional societies only to be degraded by institutions and businesses. Professionals, according to Talcott Parsons were motivated toward performing public service and good work, a view that (with respect to physicians) was apparently undermined in the 1960s and subsequent decades having first been codified by professional societies to impose some aspect of ministry on those who had not developed it individually. The view insisted, at least, on a unique relation between physician and patient, based on an explicit and professionally guaranteed moral foundation of shared expectations and valued collegial recognition more than on financial gain.

In what follows we will explore some of the behavior and attitudes of the groups and individuals in the medical community and some of the problems that result often as a reflection of changing social attitudes and changing economic pressures.

HOSPITALS

Hospitals, like physicians, may be concerned chiefly with primary care, or may be specialty facilities. They are classified as primary, secondary, tertiary or quaternary hospitals according to the level of specialization offered. Third and fourth level hospitals are often associated with a medical school and serve as teaching hospitals. Often hospitals are organized in vertical chains so a given primary or secondary hospital, when a higher degree of specialization is needed, refer to a given tertiary or quaternary hospital in the table of organization. Most of my experience has been in a tertiary and quaternary setting (I am, after all, a specialist) so that is the situation with which I am most familiar and about which I will write. However, I have had some contact with primary hospitals and have great respect for them. Simple fractures, industrial injuries (the loss of a finger for example), dislocated shoulders I have seen skillfully (and compassionately) treated at primary hospitals. More complicated injuries—a dislocated elbow for example—are referred to the next level hospital at a nearby city. Still more complicated problems—a closed head injury with prolonged loss of consciousness—may be transported, on occasion by helicopter, to a major medical center often in a large metropolis. The doctors at primary hospitals are not only medically skilled but often retain the compassion and personal involvement of the old-fashioned small town practitioner. I had a call some years ago from a doctor I did not know in a small town in New Hampshire, about two hours drive from Boston. He told me of his patient with a neurological problem, asked for guidance, then wondered whether I could come up. At least five hours taken out of a busy day. I apologized and said I would like to help but really could not afford the sacrifice of time. He became stern. "Look" he said, "I've got a very sick patient. I need help. I want you to come up." How could I deny him? He was insisting on what he felt was best for his patient and would not tolerate a refusal. Of course I went; I only hope I was of some help.

One year I was invited to spend a week in Maine as a visiting professor. The plan was to spend part of each day (or sometimes a full day) at a different facility. One full day was to be at a small white clapboard hospital in a small town, staffed by a husband and wife team and two other practitioners. They were to present cases to me and I was to discuss them (at length) and to offer suggestions. They showed me an elderly woman in the late stages of what appeared to be an inherited neurodegenerative disorder. I made a precise diagnosis and gave a long, overly erudite discussion. Much later that day, in a different room, I was introduced to a middle-aged man with what I discussed as a completely different sort of neurodegenerative disease, probably inherited. A long, self-assured discussion. Only then did they tell me (with smiles) these two patients were mother and son. Rascals! You'd think I would have guessed for previously I had been caught in the same trap taking Grand Rounds (not so grand when I take them) at City Hospital where I was shown separately a mother and daughter with Huntington's disease—which looked quite different in each—causing me to diagnose two separate disorders and then to have the trap sprung. In that small hospital in Maine they showed me an ambulatory lobsterman whose gait interested me (a difficult neurological localization) only to have them explain that many lobstermen walked that way because of their hip boots. This man, they told me, had been admitted some months earlier with a fever and a stiff neck. They recovered a yeast from his spinal fluid, treated him with a powerful drug that caused his kidneys to shut down, treated his renal failure, cured him and sent him back to lobstering. "Would you like to comment?" they queried. "You bet," I said, hoping they did not expect a long academic discussion. "Congratulations. We couldn't have done as well in Boston." I have often thought if my terminal illness requires hospitalization I'd like to go to that hospital in New Hampshire or that small white clapboard "cottage" in Maine.

The role of the visiting professor reminds me of an anecdote, perhaps apocryphal, about the Regius Professor of Medicine at Oxford who felt a social responsibility to visit periodically small outlying hospitals. On one such occasion the Houseman, (the British equivalent of our Resident) presented a patient with gastrointestinal symptoms. At the conclusion of the presentation the Professor, as was his custom, asked the Houseman what he thought the diagnosis was. "I believe sir," said the Resident "it's a simple case of indigestion". Now the Regius Professor was a stickler for accuracy of medical terminology and indigestion was not a medical term. "Indigestion" he said. "Indigestion. I don't believe I know what that means." At which the patient in the next bed remarked "And 'e calls 'imself a specialist".

Hospitals have personalities; each hospital has a distinct personality. Hospital personalities determine staff behavior and patient characteristics, and staff behavior and patient characteristics help determine hospital personality. Perhaps the outstanding determinants are the cultural characteristics of the founding and supporting organization. Towns and cities, churches and religious organizations, philanthropic agencies and now for profit businesses all participate. Doctor founded clinics have been absorbed to become part of the hospital culture. Though the science may be the same from hospital to hospital, the style of presenting it is very different.

Some personality characteristics are common to all hospitals; they pervade the medical side of the hospital community, its professional and nonprofessional staff. Perhaps this is not unique to medicine; perhaps it is evident in all so called service industries. But the kind of service offered by the medical community has a presumed moral aspect, an old fashioned idea that may no longer exist, for we are told by the French philosopher Alain Badiou "Morality is a residue of the old world" ("The Century" quoted in the New York Review October 23, 2008). It is not inherent in a fast food or other type of restaurant, which is the prototype service industry. A good waiter is supposed to *serve* yet be unobtrusive (forlorn hope) but it is a different type of service from that of a hospital employee whose job (one would hope) is to help. Yet what obtrudes are arrogance and the need to control. From the Admitting Office, where you may be kept waiting for long periods while the Admitting Officer talks with a colleague about her social life, then disinterestedly asks personal questions mainly concerned with insurance coverage, to the new doctor who hurriedly confronts you, for you must understand he is a very busy, very important man. Among the worst are the doctors' private secretaries, who control access and want you to realize they are in charge. It is those who deal with patients in a one to one relationship who are most guilty, yet nurses—as a generality—are humble, concerned, and helpful. They serve in the spirit of Abigail Adams: "If we do not lay out ourselves in the service of mankind whom should we serve?" An attitude from another time.

Case managers are another example. Previously called social workers they have been verbally elevated from the role of worker to the level of management. Once concerned with post-discharge conditions—home care, food, welfare and the like—they are now involved primarily with getting the patient out of the hospital as fast as possible so the hospital will not be financially penalized. Their disinterest in the patient despite their active involvement must be offensive to some of the more sensitive patients The transition from social worker concerned with the financial problems of the patient to case manager concerned with the financial problems of the hospital is but one more ironic reflection of changing social attitudes. As is the term case manager—the manager of a case—not a supporter of a patient. One definition of a case is a container, so the patient becomes not a person, but a container of a disease. Once again, emphasis is on treatment of a disease and not on care of a patient.

The founding and supporting agency of a hospital represents a community. The community may be geographic, religious, or social.

Often the hospital serves that community as in the case of a town or a city. Other times the community may be dispersed; for example, the founding community may be religious but the hospital non-denominational. Still, the culture of the denomination permeates the hospital and influences decisions, attitudes, and behavior. Tertiary hospitals tend to cater to a dispersed community, primary hospitals to a geographic location. Financial support for the tertiary hospital may come in part from local philanthropies (including corporations), former patients, affiliated medical schools, indirect costs included in research grants and, of course, insurance companies. This is a much less cohesive community than a city neighborhood or a town. But even for these, as society changes, the sense of "our hospital" disappears. When I was in training at City Hospital, nurses coming off the 3-11 PM shift could walk the long block to the subway without fear. These were "our nurses"; the community protected them. No longer. That was an era when the hospital provided free care to the impoverished neighborhood. The hospital took care of the community so the community took care of their nurses. Now, "We pay so you pay" is the attitude. The change from public and charity support of a charitable function is reflected in the dictionary definition of "hospital". The second edition of Webster's New International Dictionary, published in 1938 defines hospital as "An institution or place in which patients or injured persons are given medical or surgical care, *often in whole or in part at public expense or by charity*"(emphasis added). The third edition of Webster, published in 1968, gives the verbatim definition but omits the italicized phrase. The disappearance of the State Psychiatric Hospitals is emblematic of this change, a result of and a contribution to a major social upheaval. For almost a century, these institutions had served as a shelter for the socially inadequate. Not only shelter in the physical sense—for they provided housing, food, clothes and warmth—but also in the emotional sense. Despite their inadequacies and occasional brutalities, life on the inside was better than life on the outside The turmoil of the 60's, the writings of Foucault, the ideas of Laing and the 'antipsychiatrists' may have originated from a different philosophic source than the changes going on in general medicine but the effect on hospitals was the same. The social responsibility of the hospital and the responsibility of society to the hospitals were destroyed. In this sense, the deconstructionists were destructionists, and the return of patients to the community (as if the community would take care of them outside of a formal organized structured setting) was an immoral act perhaps generated by economic considerations rather than a lofty new philosophy. And while the changes in the General Hospital were not as brusque and perhaps should not be termed immoral, hospital stays were ruthlessly shortened, patient care was redefined, and economics replaced what might be called philosophy (or at least a moral outlook) as the determinant of policy.

The restructuring of hospitals, largely conditioned by economic factors, not only led to mergers and amalgamations but also to changed attitudes, goals, and behavior of hospital administrators. More than one thousand hospitals in the United States merged during the 1990s. "Care of the patient" remained the stated determinant of hospital performance but the care of the patient became secondary to making money. The role of the nurse changed. Nurse-patient relationship was diluted if not entirely destroyed. Nurse morale suffered, frustration and disillusionment led to declining numbers, and nurses' strikes—an inconceivable performance not so very long ago—jeopardized patient care. Mergers increased hospital size and administrators salaries (600 beds and close to one million dollars a year respectively as examples). One Boston Hospital, which reported a projected deficit of 175 million dollars, reimbursed its Administrator 1.35 Million in salary and benefits plus 3.5 million in deferred compensation. In addition she received $917,497 for her position on the Board of Directors of three scientific-pharmacological corporations. Using $150 as an acceptable charge for an initial office visit to a doctor in the Boston area, her hospital compensation alone could finance more than 32,000 doctor visits. Increased annual research funding was closed to seventy five million dollars in one case. Throughout the cultural clashes, the turmoil of reorganization, the loss of nurses, and the decline of morale, the hospitals continue to emphasize verbally a mission of providing the best of "warm, personalized medical care and considerate service" (Business Wire Oct 1, 1996)

The culture of the founding and supporting group pervades, even in the absence of direct participation. I used to teach at a Catholic Hospital. Quiet, cleanliness, and discipline prevailed. Nuns, in their white habits, sleeves rolled up, were constantly mopping the floors. They watched everything to be certain it was done properly. My major affiliation was with a Methodist Hospital, founded by the Deaconesses in the closing years of the 19th century. As the psychiatrist who interviewed me at the time of my staff application remarked, "We are a Methodist hospital but you don't have to be a Methodist to be on the staff". What that meant was that certain behavior patterns were taken for granted. Much of the interactions were based on implicit indications and on indirection. Not everything had to be said. There were expectations to be fulfilled without verbalization. How different from the

Jewish Hospital just down the street (I was also on the staff there) where everything was expressed, everything was explicit. When the two hospitals amalgamated for financial reasons there was a clash of cultures (although not everyone recognized it as such) sufficient to result in an article in The New Republic. The author, a staff member at the Jewish Hospital, wrote that at his hospital things had always been done in the open over a bagel and a cup of coffee, while at the other hospital things had been done in secret. Actually, things were not done in secret; everyone knew without it being stated. To my amusement, this difference in style became evident when after the consolidation of the two hospitals the signs in the Methodist Hospital office building elevators were changed. For many years a small, inconspicuous sign, the color of the elevator interior read: "Patient confidentiality is respected at all times by the Hospital Staff". If you thought about it, the things that were important were that: 1-It was a sign. That meant it had a message 2-That message was being displayed in the confined space of an elevator so it had something to do with the elevator 3-Those elevators transported doctors, nurses, other hospital personnel, patients and families 4-The message was not the same for the professional staff as it was for the public. Patients and family must have thought, "How lucky we are to have our confidences in the care of an ethical professional staff". For the professional staff it said, "Don't talk shop in elevators." After the amalgamation new large white bold-faced signs appeared: "Information about patients is confidential and should never be discussed in public places. Thank you for being considerate of our patients and their families and respecting their right to privacy." Patients and family must now have thought they were at the mercy of an unethical and talkative staff, which needed to be cautioned not to talk in public places. The implicit but understood code of behavior was now overt; the reminder was not only expressed; it was shouted in bold-faced type. This distinction permeated all activities of the new hospital complex and although a new culture is emerging (with the associated loss of some of the supporting communities) much of value has been lost.

For a hospital to function it must have a medical staff. For a doctor, affiliation with a hospital is an important asset. So, the relation between a doctor and a hospital is one of mutual benefit. In the beginning, staff doctors were often independent practitioners. Over time, an increasing number became full time hospital staff, often affiliated with a medical school leading to a two level system colloquially termed "Town and Gown". In the days of community support, open wards and free beds, the charity patients were cared for by the academic teaching services and the private patients, in private or semiprivate rooms were cared for by private practitioners. Now the open ward and the free bed have all but disappeared and the independent private practitioner has been absorbed into hospital departments, Health Maintenance Organizations or incorporated Group Practices.

Important teaching hospitals—hospitals often affiliated with a medical school—at which young doctors are trained, define themselves as having three major functions: 1—patient care 2—teaching 3—research. How carefully are these functions monitored by the Hospital Administration, and how qualified is the Hospital Administration, occupied as it is with financial matters, to assess these functions? Patient care means considerably more than medical outcome. Medical outcome may be good but patient care negligent. Alternatively, patients may die cared for and comfortable. A tough old nurse, who took care of a ward full of indigent men at City Hospital for many years, developed pneumonia. She did not have a doctor and turned to me. I called a colleague, an internist, who admitted her to the private hospital at which we both served. I kept an eye on her progress as her as fever persisted despite aggressive treatment. Early one morning I arrived to find her rumpled bed drenched from a nocturnal sweat. "Grace, why didn't you ask to have your sheets changed?" I asked. 'Do my men have to ask me to have their sheets changed?" she replied. She knew how to care for the sick. She never showed it to them—she was tough—but she cared. Things were done well; she cared for her patients in both senses of the word.

Can this be taught? Not without a major shift in societal attitudes. "Jane" shouts a young nurse down the corridor. "207 needs a bedpan". How to explain to that nurse: 1—you don't shout 2—207 is a person with a name 3—the bed pan is needed now 4—it can be brought just as well by a nurse as by Jane the 'aid'. Contrast this with the old and distinguished professor of medicine I encountered one evening carrying a cup of tea toward a patient's room. "You shouldn't have to do that "I said, "You should be practicing medicine". "I am practicing medicine," he said very gently to me.

It is hard to be sick and good patient care means doing everything possible to make it easier. But the thrust is toward greater efficiency. Patient care cannot be efficient; other aspects of the hospital should be, although much of the hospital still retains the wasteful procedures of the past. Our hospitals solicit management consultants to teach us how to take care of patients. By the very nature of their function they cannot do that. Hillary, a young member of one such consultation firm came to interview me, as the firm did with all heads of departments, to "get my input". Hillary was a vibrant, energetic young woman who exuded health. I am sure she had never been seriously ill. "It's hard to be sick" I told her "and when we are well we forget just how hard it is". I explained the role of the doctor, in my judgement, was to make it easier for the patient to cope with the illness. In due time a very thick volume appeared—a management consultants report. My contribution was summarized briefly. "Dr. Locke believes medicine is a cottage industry".

I am afraid the role of patient care in the broad sense is beyond retrieval. Our hospitals give good medical and surgical treatment; patients often get better, go into remission or gain time, but caring for the patient has disappeared. This was summarized at one hospital at which I worked that distributed yellow smiley face lapel pins to its nursing staff to be worn on the uniform chest. These pins would serve as surrogates and save the trouble of a real smile.

The second function—teaching—is a complicated area. Teaching generally means House Staff—interns and residents—although medical students may be included. Interns and residents are a major component of the hospital staff and constitute a serious recruitment problem. A large teaching hospital may have upward of one hundred House Staff. To get adequate recruits—both quantity and quality—requires certain criteria. Salary and work schedule are important but most important is the satisfaction of the current House Staff for its members serve as the major advertisement to attract new interns. Often applicants have friends on the current staff. Even if not, House Staff can be trusted to tell it "like it is". If they feel overworked, abused or disgruntled the applicant pool may diminish. So they must be treated carefully. Do not demand too much, do not reprimand, be gentle. Once again, how different from the way it was. When I was in training, Intern meant within the walls. You lived in, had every second night on duty and earned ten dollars a month. You served the hospital in exchange for an opportunity to learn. And Residents too (the year after internship) as the name suggests were resident on their on call nights. No longer. Now you can take call from home. You live out and that requires a substantial salary. Residents are a carefully treated privileged group. And so, when I was approached by the Chief Resident to increase the number of Neurology teaching sessions I said I'd be happy to. "We could meet on given mornings at 7AM in the Cafeteria. "We can't do that," said the Chief Resident; "we don't start until 8".

Lack of student interest makes teaching a burden. Teaching time is a contribution one makes. It is uncompensated time away from a busy schedule, except for the compensation provided by the enthusiastic student.

When there is no interest it is a chore. So, I reported to our assigned meeting room one Thursday morning at 11 o'clock. The room was empty; the House Staff had not yet showed up. At about 11:10 a fourth year student arrived. The custom was for a case—a patient currently in the hospital—to be presented *in absentia* for discussion. We waited for about five minutes for three House Officers to drift in. "Who has the case?" I asked. No one was prepared. Options: 1—cancel and return to my office and catch up on some outstanding obligations 2—try to salvage the situation and use the remaining part of the hour to teach. "Well," I said, "I'll tell you about a patient I saw this morning at the Diabetic Unit. I described a man with a painful shoulder. He had undiagnosed Parkinson's disease one manifestation of which is loss of associated movements. The lack of normal arm swing when walking causes the shoulder to "freeze up" and become painful. Perhaps I could make a single point for them to take away. A sore shoulder might mean consider Parkinson's disease. "What do you think?" I asked. A young woman, perhaps struck by the fact I had seen the patient on the Diabetic Unit, said "Diabetic amyotrophy". Diabetic amyotrophy is characterized by a painful, tender thigh in elderly diabetic men, and it just happened that I had written one of the early articles on the disorder, with two colleagues. "Oh" I said, "I didn't know diabetic amyotrophy affects the arm" "Of course it does" said the resident. "Where did you learn that?" I asked. "It says so in Harrison's text book" she replied. "Let's look it up," I suggested. "Would you get Harrison from the Nursing station?" which was just across the hall. "That's making busy work" she replied. "But we should be sure. Please get the book". Reluctantly she went, reluctantly she looked it up, and reluctantly she conceded there was no mention of pain in the shoulder. "I've got to take the book back" she said as she left the room, not to return. I don't know if I made my point about shoulder pain and Parkinsons disease. I do know I generated an entry into my personnel file that "Locke berates the House Staff". Perhaps I should have been more gentle. Certainly it might have better conveyed information. But would it have better dealt with the arrogance?

No matter. This was only didactic teaching. But teaching also takes place outside of designated hours at the bedside in relation to flesh and blood patients. One Tuesday in June I was asked to see a woman admitted on Thursday because of weakness of the legs. June is the end of the academic year. The interns have a year of real life experience, their residents two. The patient was an obese diabetic—esthetically unattractive. Examination revealed what was suspected (and later confirmed) to be a herniated fifth cervical disc—a curable disorder. "Why didn't you call me earlier?" I asked the House Staff when the neurosurgeon decided that it was too late to operate. "We were waiting for the CT scan to see if she had a stroke" the resident replied. Now a stroke on one side of the brain affects the opposite side of the body. A disorder of spinal cord affects both sides. This was June. Had my teaching been that ineffective? But this fundamental fact was also taught in Medical School. The delay caused the patient to lose use of her legs, control of her bladder and bowels and to be confined to a dependent life with early death probable. I thought this important enough to call to the attention of the physician in charge of House Staff training. "Well" he said, "we'll have to look into it." I thought their noses ought to be rubbed in it so they would never forget but that would alienate our charges and ultimately diminish our applicant pool. I suspect nothing was ever done about it.

It is easy enough to teach facts and facts are treated as the core of medical education. They can be assessed as knowledge on paper and pencil tests. But facts are not what makes a doctor. Facts can be looked up in books. A colleague, checking a fact in a book was asked by his patient who was present at the time "Doctor, do you have to look it up in a book?" He simply replied, "Would you prefer that I don't?" The quality of a doctor is determined by behavior not by knowledge of facts. So, I roused an Intern at six one morning to tell him I thought the woman he had asked me to see had meningitis, and needed a spinal tap. Meningitis, an infection of the coverings of the brain, is often curable if treatment is started early and may be permanently destructive if treatment is delayed. Diagnosis and decision about type of treatment (that is, choice of antibiotic) requires a spinal tap and examination of the spinal fluid. I asked the Intern to perform the tap (as is customary) and to telephone me just as soon as he had results. When, at 10:30 I still had not heard I phoned him and asked what the tap had shown. "I haven't done it yet" he said. "Why not?" I asked. "I want to talk it over with the team at our 11 o'clock meeting" he said. "Why?" I asked. "To dilute the responsibility," he replied. Taking responsibility is a prime attribute of a physician; that's what the practice of medicine is all about. But I cannot teach behavior and young doctors would be resentful should I try. As would the hospital authorities for it would undermine our competitive status in the arena of House Staff applications.

Furthermore, there is always litigation. A patient was admitted to the hospital in the middle of the night. The on call doctor was notified but did not get out of bed. On rounds, in the morning, the patient was dead, never having been seen by a doctor. I said to the Chief, about the resident, a bright young man with an MDPhD combination "We should fire him"

"If we do" said the Chief "he'll sue". I cannot be sanctimonious about his response; the stone must remain uncast. When Neurology Boards still entailed examination of patients I served as an examiner present while a candidate took a history and examined a patient. I watched him measure the blood pressure in each arm and do a careful, thorough examination. When he presented his findings he neglected to tell me the blood pressures. They were crucial to the diagnosis for they were strikingly different on the two sides, leading to restricted blood flow on one side of the brain, and to the neurological diagnosis. In an effort to be helpful, and to direct him to the correct conclusion I said "I noticed you took the blood pressure in each arm, What did you find?" "It was normal," he said. "Give me the figures," I requested. "120/80 on both sides" he said. His presentation had been good, his examination had been thorough, his diagnosis, though incorrect, was consistent with his presentation and was logically achieved. He was a competent neurologist. But he had lied. I said to the Chief Examiner "I would like to fail this man because he lied" "Do whatever you think proper," said the Chief Examiner, "but I know this man and I know if you fail him he'll sue you". What a dilemma. I had my principles but here was reality. I had neither the time nor the emotional energy to be sued. The Board did not indemnify us. The candidate was not a bad physician. He might miss diagnoses but probably no more then most of us. I passed him. I worry about it to this day but who knows what life would have been like had I failed him.

One who does know is the Chief of another Neurology service, a man of principle, who had among his trainees a young resident who was apparently negligent and incompetent. The Professor discussed the situation with the trainee and outlined the areas that needed improvement. Improvement did not occur and so, when the time for reappointment to the subsequent year of the training program arrived, the young man was passed over. He sued. My colleague, fortunately indemnified by the University, pursued the situation to its conclusion, thereby eliminating his contribution to the medical community of an incompetent doctor. But the trainee almost certainly found other ways to end up practicing despite investment of time and energy by a principled colleague.

The third hospital function—research—has the least effect on the personality of the hospital, its doctors, and its patients, perhaps because it is often conducted out of sight. It may be basic, it may be clinical, and its major effect is to generate money for the hospital (as well as for the investigator), often through what is termed "indirect costs" of a grant. Funds may be provided to the hospital by the grant or may be redistributed from the associated medical school. The presence of the research investigators may contribute to the intellectual climate of the hospital and certainly to its prestige. The topic of clinical investigation introduces two additional considerations: 1—the Internal Review Board 2—Informed consent. Each hospital must have an Internal Review Board composed of physicians from various disciplines, a member of the community (perhaps a clergyman) and if possible a bioethicist. Its function is to review ethical issues, protect patients, and to a lesser extent make scientific decisions. Some hospitals have a Clinical Research Center supported by a Government Program Grant to the hospital, with oversight by a Scientific Advisory Committee which reviews protocols for proposed research and passes judgement on such things as the importance of the project, the safety to participants, the relevance of the procedures to the proposed objective, ethical considerations and suitability of the hospital to the undertaking. Conflict of interest is not eliminated; the proposal may potentially generate substantial income for the hospital; the protocol may come from an Advisory Committee member's own department. A colleague may have spoken to a member and lobbied for approval.

The issue of informed consent is broader for it applies not only to research participants but also to patients undergoing almost any sort of procedure, no matter how benign. It should not be a *pro forma* undertaking: is the patient given enough time to read the document? Is the language understandable? Are the implications clear? Does the patient know what the document being signed really means? And the inclusion of all potential catastrophes, no matter how remote, makes the document frightening. Were I to take seriously all the considerations I read in an informed consent document I would never sign one. The real question, however, is whether any patient, no matter how knowledgeable, no matter how much information is provided, can make a truly "informed" decision. Better to chose your doctor with care, and then trust her—if, that is, you are given the chance to choose your doctor, and then having done so, that doctor is allowed to stay with you.

Which brings us to the topic of Hospitalists. These are young physicians—often recent graduates of training programs—employed by the hospital or its professional organization to be responsible for all patients admitted to the hospital medical service. On the surgical side, Physicians Assistants perform a similar function. Upon a patients admission the hospitalist becomes the doctor of record. This means that your own doctor who (presumably) knows all about you—your likes, your desires, your allergies, your emotional needs, your past history—is no longer taking care of you. The good side of this system is that the hospitalist works long hours (often 12 hours a day for a week at a stretch followed by a week off) and is there when needed. A second hospitalist—a nocturnist—takes the night shift. The bad side is that decisions are being made about a disease or disorder, not about a patient. But that's the way the business is run, and business it is. For it generates income for the hospital.

Other aspects of business permeate hospitals. They now advertise—in the Yellow Pages and on radio and television. They have diversified investments in retirement homes and assisted living facilities. They close their nursing schools and non-remunerative hospital departments. They try to balance the books with charitable appeals but remain administratively top heavy with upper echelon officers receiving annual salaries of the order or one million dollars. Years ago, the academic worth of a hospital was judged by potential interns on the basis of how deep in the red was the institution. The more in debt the greater its academic prestige. Remnants of other old-fashioned ideas persist. Women's auxiliaries still have plant sales and run the gift or thrift shop at the hospital, the proceeds of which will buy an important piece of operating room equipment or other property. And since patients constitute the major source of income, giving ambulance drivers the occasional bottle of whisky will help them decide to bring patients to your Emergency Room rather than to the hospital just down the street.

While trying to run the hospital as a business much of the internal organization is unbusinesslike—left over from the old (and unyielding) culture. My experience with it comes from the electroencephalography laboratory I set up at the hospital. The procedure was: 1—the test was ordered and scheduled 2—transportation department was called and asked to get the patient. Often there was a delay—no transporter was available, the patient was in the bathroom, a doctor was with the patient, some other cause 3—the patient was brought to the lab where the technician applied the electrodes to the scalp while the machine continued to stand idle. 4—the technician performed the test and then removed the electrodes and cleaned the scalp of the electrode paste. 5—Transportation was called to return the patient to the floor. 6—the procedure was repeated for the next patient. How much better to assign one transporter full time to the EEG department. The patient could be brought to the lab well in advance. The transporter, following suitable training, could apply the electrodes. Then, while the technician performed the test, the transporter could get and prepare the next patient. While the second patient was being tested, the transporter could remove the electrodes and clean the scalp, then return patient #1 to the floor, and without returning to the lab collect the third patient. That way the down time for the expensive EEG machine would be minimized. Would the EEG technician feel overworked? I suggested a base monthly salary for a given number of records performed—amount of salary and number of records to be determined by the administration from past performance. Any additional records would be compensated on a prearranged fee per record determined by the administration. This would provide the technicians with incentive, the hospital with greater daily income from the EEG laboratory and the patient might profit from a shorter hospital stay. The administration, to which I proposed this found the plan unacceptable.

Hospital Departments could be considered as the interface between the hospital limb and the medical limb of the three-legged medical community. They are headed by doctors, often professors at an affiliated medical school, and are committed to their staff at the same time they are committed to the hospital. This ambiguous position calls for an even minded, impartial individuals who can deal with sectarian problems in a fair way. The hospital provides space, furniture, equipment, and often financial support (perhaps redistributed from the medical school). The Department supplies staff members, their patients, grants, knowledge, and prestige. The distinction at the interface of what is hospital and what is doctor is often blurred—more so for the Chief with his divided interest than for his junior staff.

The Professor—the Department Chief—is a different kind of individual now a days. He must be a pragmatist, concerned with money as much as with intellectual property. And professors have proliferated in part because salary, provided by the department, is determined by academic level. So, the department in which I trained sixty years ago had one professor then and at least ten professors now. In part, this is because if individuals raise the endowment to support them—which will persist long after their departure—they can have the professorship. Much like grade inflation in universities, the grade "Professor" no longer signifies what it should. As has been pointed out, the star system no longer exists (just like in the movies). When I was still in the early stages of my career the distinction between Chief and others was clear. I was not Assistant Chief when I was second in command; I was Chief Assistant and never allowed to forget it.

The Chief of Department sets the tone for the whole department by behavior. The negligent, unconcerned Chief focused only on his own research has a negligent, unconcerned staff. During my training, there was a period in the second year when the resident was responsible for consultations in the rest of the hospital. Each month a specified senior staff member served as back up on whom the resident could call if faced with a major clinical problem. The Professor, along with other members of the senior staff accepted this role. One was always reluctant to call the senior staff during the night but sometimes good care required it. Should the need arise to call the Professor when he was on service it was always done with trepidation. A sleepy professor answered the phone, heard the problem, and invariably said, "Would you like me to come in?" That question, which could usually be answered in the negative—all you needed was advice—did more to set the tone of the department and to govern future behavior—to give you a role model—than lectures or textbooks. This man accepted his responsibility and by doing so taught me to accept mine. Do they still make such doctors?

In the expected course of events, the Professor had to retire. A new professor had to be selected. A Search Committee was formed, appointed by the Dean of the Medical School. It included the professors of Medicine and Surgery at the hospital to protect the hospital's interests and a professor of Neurology from another hospital to protect the interests of the Medical School Department of Neurology. They asked to interview me, as I was now the Acting Director of the Unit and had been there for a long time. I knew its strengths and weaknesses, its needs and goals. I could offer them advice and guidance they said. We met in a small conference room. They began by thanking me for taking the time to help them. The Professor of Surgery told me of his proposal to appoint a neurosurgeon from another hospital as our new professor of neurology despite the fact these were distinct disciplines. The Professor of Medicine countered with a plan of his own. The neurologist was cautious in his comments for it was not in his interest to allow a dominant distinguished individual become head of a competing department. I listened to their discussion, which lasted about an hour, at the end of which they thanked me for my help. While the search, which took several years, was going on, my staff was disseminated, attracted by other departments of Neurology, some of which were in our own university. The uncertainty was demoralizing and made it impossible to maintain a cohesive group. One subsequent search, when our professorship became vacant again, took seven years to complete. The Search Committee was rarely convened for it was not in the interest of the Committee Chairman to have a new professor installed.

Professor's behaviors are determined all too often by non-professorial aspects of character. Ego—an important attribute in driving them toward professorships—enters into decisions and attitudes, and may interfere with the alleged function of a professor—to nurture students and to disseminate knowledge. Like politicians, who, driven by ego needs, are the least fit to govern in the interest of the public, so professors driven by ego needs are also the least fit to profess. But there are outstanding exceptions. As a resident on the consultation service—over fifty years ago—I was called to see a patient on the medical ward. As I started my examination, the Professor of Medicine accompanied by a half dozen House Staff converged on the patient. I introduced myself (it was early in the academic year) and said I would come back later, when they had completed their round. "No" said the Professor "we will come back later when you have completed your examination and you will teach us about the diagnosis". Amazing. Many years later, as a young neurologist, I would take a monthly conference at the VA hospital to which the professor had retired. To my surprise, he invariably attended. These were clinical conferences in which a patient, diagnosis unknown to the discussant, was presented and the case analyzed. At the end of one conference I approached him and said, "I am honored that you come to these things but I cannot help but wonder why" "I have always been interested in the way another person thinks," he said. A real professor.

But at another conference, a brain cutting, the situation was different. Here the case of an autopsied patient is presented and discussed from the floor starting with the most junior member and ending with the professor; then the brain is cut allowing determination of accuracy of each diagnosis. Once I arrived late, so found a seat in the back of the room. One after another, the House Staff and junior Staff discussed a temporal lobe lesion. Next to last, I offered an argument for a different location. The professor, who came next, was confronted by a dilemma; which to choose? Go with House Staff or take a different tack? He chose the House Staff and diagnosed a temporal lobe lesion. As the brain was sliced, my location, on the medial aspect of the hemisphere proved correct. "MY GOD, HE'S RIGHT," said the professor loud enough for me to hear from his seat in the front row. I knew at that moment I had lost my job supervising residents, a conclusion confirmed two or three months later.

At one time, the ambiguity of the departments—hospital or doctor—created the dichotomy of Town and Gown. Private facilities were distinguished from wards, private patients from ward patients. Some hospitals were entirely private, often without a House Staff in the very early days. Some were entirely House Staff and entirely ward with senior staff supervisors; municipal hospitals were an example. Some hospitals had both divisions. But with the era of monetization, the distinction began to disappear. All patients were now private because all patients became a source of hospital income. Former ward patients on subsequent hospitalization were assigned private doctors who had never seen them before and might never see them again. And with that change the concept of "on service" evolved. A physician in a given department was on service for a specified period—let's say a month. What that means is that were I to admit you to hospital as my patient (something that is more and more difficult to do for in most cases you would have a hospitalist assigned as your doctor) and should I feel the need for advice from a consultant in specialty area, I could no longer choose the specific physician I desired but would have to accept the consultant on service for that month. My desire for a specific colleague might reflect my sense that that individual's personality would work well with yours. Or it might reflect my awareness of a special strength or skill—an oncologist with a particular interest in cancer of the breast or an infectious disease specialist with extensive experience treating tuberculosis as examples. But my chosen colleague might not be on service that month and were I to insist the on service consultant might be offended.

Which brings up the role of the consultant in the contemporary hospital. In the past, the consultant was expected to offer an opinion not a procedure. The procedure or treatment by the consultant could be obtained at the request of the referring doctor but it was your doctor who was in charge. On occasion, the consultant might be asked to become the doctor of record. On other occasion, the consultant might be asked to participate in parallel with your doctor. Frequently your own doctor would implement the suggestions of the consultant. My practice as a consultant was always to send a detailed letter to the referring physician outlining my findings, my conclusions, and my recommendations for the referring physician to implement or not. On one occasion at the end of an office visit I told the patient my conclusions and my recommendations. He said, "Thank you doctor, but I would like to talk it over with Dr. Brown first." I said "Of course. I plan to send Dr Brown a complete report and let him decide with you how to proceed." He said, "Let me tell you why, so you will not think I do not value your opinion. One morning I waked and knew there was something wrong. I didn't have a doctor, so I went down the alphabetical list in the Yellow Pages looking for a doctor near me. Dr. Brown was the first one I found. I phoned him, he came over, examined me, and said, "I think you're having a GI bleed. I believe you should go to the hospital. May I call an ambulance?" I said "Yes". When the ambulance came, he got in and rode with me to hospital, and stayed by my side until he was sure I was in safe hands and the situation was under control. Then he had to make his way back to my house, get his car, and start on his daily rounds. I don't do a thing without talking with Dr. Brown first." They don't make them like that anymore.

A gastrointestinal hemorrhage is an acute emergency; patients may exsanguinate very quickly. The responsible physician stands by until the patient is stable. Therefore, you can imagine my surprise when a young resident dealing with an acute GI bleed said, "Well, it's five o'clock. I'm off duty" and he left. How to deal with that type of situation? As a supervisor, you have no disciplinary procedures available. At one stage my departmental assignment, paid for by departmental funds, was to supervise the residents. We met first thing each morning to review the admissions of the previous day. The rules were that the admitting resident of the day work up every patient admitted before five o'clock; patients who arrived after five were the responsibility of the resident on night duty. One morning from the list of admissions there was one patient whom nobody knew. She had not been examined; there was no work up. "What time did she come in?" I asked. "4:30" I was told. "Who was on days yesterday?" I asked. "I was" said one young man. "You were responsible to admit until five o'clock," I said. "That's not the way I define my duty," he said. I could have replied that I was the one to define duties but it would have done no good. The law of retributive justice required that when he went on to become a Professor and Chief at a prestigious medical school (as he did) he would have to deal with similar arrogance and presumption. But perhaps he didn't care, for by then standards had declined even further

DOCTORS

As is evident, the distinction between the role of doctors and of hospitals is not clear cut and it becomes less clear as hospitals assume more medical functions by delegating them to hospital staff. Doctors willingly relinquish responsibilities and duties to hospitals because of the structure of the reimbursement system. Hospitals may pay salaries that range up to about $400,000 a year for young surgeons. Once the responsibility of the physician was to the patient who reimbursed him, (physicians were mostly men in that era) and to the patient who did not reimburse him because that was the ethic of the period. It was an honor to be requested to donate a half day a week to a free clinic and a privilege to do so. It had its rewards: interesting diagnoses, grateful patients, and occasionally homemade cookies. One distinguished neurosurgeon, a Boston Brahmin, who would rap the knuckles of his assistants at the operating table, once remarked to me "Locke, I like poor patients and I like sick patients and the poorer they are and the sicker they are the more I like them." Now there are no free clinics and there are no poor patients in terms of reimbursement. The physician is removed from the financial aspects (someone else does the billing) and payments come from the insurance industry, including the government. The physician's responsibility now is to the insurer; the patient is an accessory. The important thing now is to use the right reimbursement code. A gynecologist asked me to see a woman because of headache. In those days, referrals were made doctor to doctor; now a days you tell the patient to call—it saves time. I sent him a report and filed an insurance claim with a narrative as well as the coded diagnosis. The claim was denied. I called and explained that in the judgement of the referring doctor a consultation was necessary. "What was the diagnosis?" asked the young High School graduate who denied the claim. "Headache" I told her. "You shooda wrote severe headache" she said.

The ethic of that bygone period was a work ethic and one of personal responsibility. "Why don't you go home?" a colleague asked me late one evening; "I saw you on the wards at six this morning." "In which case" I replied, "you should go home too". Doctors wrote patients letters summarizing their findings, conclusions and suggestions. They maintained a professional relationship despite difficulties. "I've let that woman abuse me for almost 40 years" said one colleague about a patient he had asked me to see. Another said to an abusive patient "Remember, I didn't make you sick but I will do all I can to make you better." In general, my colleagues were good people, motivated by a sense of duty, a desire to help, and a devotion to their profession. Of course, they made mistakes and yes they worked for money but that was not the underlying motivation. And they had individual personalities, which influenced many aspects of their practices—their specialties, their treatments and the kinds of patients they attracted. An old maid of a doctor (despite the fact that he was a married man with a family) took care of a large number of elderly women. He also took care of young girls by arrangement with a nearby private school that attracted teen-agers from all over the country. He asked me to see one of the girls who had come to see hem because of headaches. She was easy to talk to so we chatted about irrelevancies for a long time—music, the social scene, life in Boston. Finally, we got around to the headaches. I asked her to tell me about them. She said they usually occurred when she was popping speed. "Did you tell that to Dr. Olmaid?" I asked. "What him?" she answered, "he wouldn't understand." A doctor's personality enters into many nonmedical aspects of the relationship with a patient that ultimately may affect the medical diagnosis or decision. And the relationship is usually established on the basis of personality—either implied or expressed—and the mood of the moment, not on medical grounds. A harried physician, a worried physician, a physician with family problems or other intrusions into daily life is, in some ways as impaired as a physician with a drug dependency. All of these interfere with clarity of diagnostic thinking and with performance. Diagnosis starts with the relationship. The patient must be won over; trust must be established. I remember a pediatrician who would ignore the four-year-old patient, talking exclusively to the mother while he played with something inapparent in his lap. Shortly enough the youngster came over to see what was going on, was allowed to play with the item—whatever it was—and before long had taken the place of the toy on the doctor's lap. Mother could then be ignored; the patient was now the doctor's.

A tricky part of the professional relationship is the doctor's emotional reaction to a patient. We are taught it should be neutral but it never is. You like some patients and not others. But beware it does not get in the way. A colleague asked me to see his wife who was having trouble keeping her footing when aboard their sailboat. He was one of three physicians I knew from old established Boston families and it showed. All three did laboratory research, more or less as a hobby, for they did not have to work. On the day of her appointment his wife was half an hour late. I was annoyed. I have always felt a doctor should be on time. If patients are kept waiting that is a sign of contempt; it says that patients do not count, that their time is not important. It also indicates the doctor does not know how to manage time, perhaps indicative of something much broader. Similarly, if a patient is late that may indicate disinterest, unwillingness to participate or even contempt.

Ordinarily when a patient is that late I explain that there is not enough time left in the assigned hour to do an adequate job and that I feel it unfair to ask other patients to wait because one patient was late. But this was George's wife and I still had half an hour. However, I was irritated by what I construed as a sense of entitlement. She never even said she was sorry to be late. A quick history was unremarkable—she was a little unsteady on the boat—and the examination unrevealing except she missed the occasional up-down when I checked position sense in the toes. Was she disinterested, unwilling to participate, did she think it was silly? In my irritation, I decided to pass it off and told her husband I was unable to diagnose an abnormality. Shortly afterwards a neighboring hospital got the first CT scanner in Boston. A spinal meningioma—a benign tumor—pressing on the tracts that transmit position sense was revealed, operation was successful, and she was cured. I had missed it because I had been irritated. My annoyance interposed itself between me and my patient. It obscured the important detail and the difference between the expert and the casual physician is in the details. Fortunately, technology prevented a major catastrophe.

Technology, however, presents problems of its own in the training of young doctors. No need to think. The scanner (or computer) will do it for you. When our hospital first got its own CT, tests had to be approved by a neurologist or by a radiologist so that the machine would not be used prodigally. A typical exchange would be for a House Officer to request a CT of brain. "Why do you want it?" "I would inquire. "To rule out a subdural hematoma" was the frequent reply. A subdural hematoma is a blood clot on the brain, frequently the result of head injury, potentially destructive and surgically curable. So, it is an important diagnosis not to miss. "Do you think he has a subdural?" I would ask. "He could have" was the type of reply. "Yes, he could have, but does he?" I would ask. "It's possible," says the reluctant House Officer, unwilling to take a stand. How can I teach these young doctors the task of a doctor is to make a diagnosis, to take a responsibility. In this situation—a definitive study to prove you right or wrong—you can do no harm to a patient. Marshall the facts; reach a conclusion; if you are correct you will have learned something; if you are incorrect you will have learned something. But if you are undecided, uncommitted, you will learn nothing. All too often, I have heard the uncommitted House Officer say, when told the results of the scan "That's what I thought". As Chaucer said (he said it better) "Naught attempted naught achieved".

This approach to technology, in a season of cost consciousness, leads to overuse and excessive expense. Take, for example, the case of an acute stroke. In the early hours following a stroke, no change in brain structure is visible on CT scan. A stroke patient newly admitted to hospital invariably had a CT of brain performed. It is read as normal and does not alter the clinical diagnosis or treatment of an obviously hemiplegic stroke. Because it was "negative", it is usually repeated a day or two later and now shows the morphology of the stroke already treated. The patient, or the insurance company, now faces the not insignificant cost of two CT scans rather than one. You might argue this results from the need to practice "defensive medicine" for the trial lawyers are lurking in the wings. That, however, is a problem for the legislatures and the courts to resolve and should not be for the hospitals and medical schools to deal with

This does lead, however, to the intrusion of the insurance companies into the practice of medicine and turns out to be a very difficult problem to resolve, for on the one hand we want to keep costs limited to what is necessary and on the other hand want to practice good medicine and not interfere with the doctor's judgement. The problem arises for many reasons. First, there are many insurance programs. Each company may offer more than one option, at varying premium rates, so patients are permitted different options. The doctor may be allowed one option (for a procedure, for example) under one program and denied that option under another. If denied, the level of practice is determined by criteria outside the medical situation of a particular patient. If permitted under the program the physician may have to request permission (on line), be required to justify the request (on line) be granted permission or told that more information is needed and be required to make an appointment to discuss (by telephone) the situation with a doctor from the insurance company. By insurance company contracts, time is costly but these ten minutes in seeking permission are neither reimbursed nor applied to patient treatment time. And it may be different for each patient and each insurance company. Often the insurance criteria for a test or procedure are not specified in advance of a request; only after the fact does the doctor learn the reasoning which may not apply to the next case. At the same time, we want to prevent the expense entailed by the ordering of unnecessary tests, often by the young inexperienced physician defensively so when questioned by the attending doctor an explanation denying responsibility will be available, supported by the negative test.

A new twist is the decision to reimburse on the basis of outcome. Outcome depends in part on the type of patient treated; the pediatrician who deals with sore throats and running noses will have patients who universally have a good outcome. The oncologist who treats patients with terminal cancer will have a patient population for whom the outcome is usually poor. Blue Cross Blue Shield of Massachusetts advertises on National Public Radio that it "believes in rewarding hospitals and doctors for the quality and outcome of the health care" they provide. Even if outcome is determined by comparison with the outcomes of a group of colleagues practicing the same specialty this is hardly a legitimate comparison. Patients differ, their complicating illnesses differ, their vulnerabilities differ. A scientific match—a so-called control group—cannot be established. Most important, outcome reflects the results of treatment, not the level of patient care. Dying patients are entitled to good care—perhaps even more than the robust convalescent—but under this insurance program patient care is not a criterion. 'What is odious in death is not death itself," said J.S. Mill "but the act of dying". In that act the patient and the family need the help that a trusted doctor can offer. A hospice, which is cheaper (and therefore more efficient), can also help, but its help is based on a new relationship—never as strong as that with the old-fashioned family doctor.

What to use in arriving at a diagnosis? It has always seemed to me that everything is up for grabs. Many of my colleagues would not agree; many, I suspect, thought my behavior strange. For starters, I would answer my own phone. If I were not available, I would get a message and call back. "Is this the doctor?" asks a startled voice. "Yes" I reply. "I didn't expect to talk with you," she says. "Then why did you call?" I ask. "Oh, I wanted to talk with you but whenever I call my own doctor I only get to talk to the secretary." Answering the phone is not without self-interest. It establishes the relationship and tells the caller what can be expected from me. It gives me information—how appropriate is the referral, how urgent is a visit. It may allow an early diagnosis or assessment of the effects of treatment; voices and articulation may be markers of disorders such as myasthenia, multiple sclerosis, and amyotrophic lateral sclerosis.

All other aspects of behavior enter into diagnosis. As I would tell my students "Life is nothing but a Rorschach test", (the biggest inkblot is your spouse). Everything about a patient gives information: dress, carriage, posture, tone of voice. The little old lady who comes into the office on minced steps, wearing a little black hat with a veil and sits stiffly on the edge of a chair tells me, before saying a word, that getting a concise, coherent history will be tough, and the history may be the most important part of the interaction. "Listen to the patient; he's telling you the diagnosis" is the old admonition. It takes time but it is worth it (financially as well as medically) for an early correct diagnosis saves a lot of unnecessary tests. Here are two illustrative cases:

A middle-aged man came to see me after having been studied at a famous but busy Boston Clinic. He wanted a second opinion about how to proceed with his recently diagnosed cerebral aneurysm. His story was that after a stressful week he had gone to his summer place on Martha's Vineyard. He was alone and said when he went to bed he suddenly developed an acute headache. He finally got to sleep, waked Saturday morning feeling better, spent a weekend in the country, drove to the ferry Sunday night, drove home, and arranged to be seen at the Clinic Monday. There he was diagnosed as having had a subarachnoid hemorrhage, underwent arteriogram, which showed two small aneurysms, and following the arteriogram had signs of a small stroke from which he gradually recovered. He was advised to have surgical repair of the aneurysms and asked my opinion. During his presentation, he kept looking at his watch and periodically would ask, "Do I still have time?" I had allotted him the usual one hour and, as he was the last patient of the day, we could run overtime if he needed it. I felt I needed more information; there was something missing. A patient with a subarachnoid hemorrhage doesn't putter about his farm for two days, then drive the long trip home, then walk into the doctor's office. "Tell me more," I requested. Slowly it came out, with frequent glances at his wristwatch. Unable to sleep Friday night, and knowing from experience that orgasm led to sleep, he had masturbated. At the moment of climax he experienced a severe headache. He had not told this to his doctors because they had been in a hurry. Aneurysms may rupture at the moment of sexual climax, but there is also a nonaneurysmal headache that may occur with sexual climax—referred to as orgasm headache. The clues, had his doctors explored the possibility, were that the headache was gone Saturday morning and that he engaged in normal, perhaps even strenuous, activity for the next three days. Ironically, he was found to have aneurysms (at the expense of a small stroke) but they were quite small,—below the size that demanded surgery—and. there was no evidence they had bled. I gave him the best information available and strongly recommended a conservative course. But the anxiety generated by his knowledge of the presence of these small aneurysms was too much for him to live with in comfort. About two months later, he called to ask a referral to a surgeon. Once again, I recommended a conservative approach and gave him the name of a group that dealt with aneurysms in the least invasive way. Had his physicians listened he might have been spared the arteriogram, its expense, the small stroke, the subsequent anxiety and the need to seek probably unnecessary surgical intervention.

A second instance relies not on history, but on an unusual observation, (everything is up for grabs). An elderly woman had been hospitalized elsewhere for a week because of tingling in the hands. During that hospitalization, she had undergone myelography—a test in which a dye is put into the spinal canal to allow visualization of the spinal cord. The test is uncomfortable, may be followed by prolonged severe headache, and like all such tests is expensive. The myelogram showed no abnormality. When she arrived at our hospital (for another disorder), I was asked to see her. I knew two things prior to my visit: 1—she was old and 2—both hands were affected. Therefore, it could not be a stroke (which would normally involve only one hand and also other parts) and it was not in upper spinal cord (the myelogram had excluded that although pernicious anemia, which affects upper spinal cord, would not show on myelogram and needed to be excluded by blood test). I arrived on the ward at about 6AM, a good time to make rounds because patients are still in their rooms, charts are in the rack, House Staff is not yet there to ask their interminable questions or utter their interminable complaints. I went into the patient's room after knocking softly. She was still asleep, her hands folded across her chest, and she was wearing gloves. White cotton gloves. What did that mean? The snug fitting gloves protected her hands from brushing directly against the bedclothes or from the movement of the bedclothes against her hands. Usually the disagreeable sensation produced by friction against the skin indicates a peripheral nerve lesion. She waked, I looked at her hands and wrists, was able to confirm my suspicion of a bilateral carpal tunnel syndrome (pressure on the median nerve at the wrist often relieved by injection or minor surgery), and told her I thought we could cure her. "If you do," she said, "I will pray for you for the rest of my life." As luck would have it she succumbed not long after (relieved of her carpal tunnel symptoms) to the leukemia which had brought her to the hospital; and no other patient has offered to pray for me since then.

Language is, of course, the most important part of human behavior in the medical relation. The medical examination is divided by the textbooks into two parts: obtaining a history and performing a physical examination. However, the history—the way it is told, the oversights, the omissions, the points of emphasis—are all as much a part of the physical examination as are listening to the chest or tapping a reflex. Language is a sensitive indicator of what is going on, if one knows how to listen. The job is one of translation. Not only do symptoms have meaning, but also the way they are described has meaning. The language of description is culture and generation bound, but one can almost always learn. I interned in St. Louis, having been educated in Boston. A frequent Chief Complaint (the Chief Complaint is a summary statement of the important symptoms) was "I got the misery". I never really knew what the misery was although the interns who had been educated in Atlanta or Nashville had no trouble with this Chief Complaint. In Boston, when talking about gait, the word "drag" means spastic and "drunk" means cerebellar (that part of the central nervous system that plays an important role in coordination).

Everything is up for grabs. I go to the waiting room to greet a new patient. Patients are scheduled an hour apart, so the waiting room is really a part of the office; the examination starts there. A well-dressed, middle-aged woman—apparently a suburbanite—and a man, I guess to be her husband, are waiting. Right away, I know something about these people, their background, their attitudes, their style. She is my patient; he is concerned, supportive, and available. They have a good relationship. I invite her in and he asks her (not me) whether she would like him to join her. Obviously, he respects her and her wishes. At her request, they both come in. After a little small talk, I ask her why she is coming to see me. "I've got foot drop," she says. Foot drop results from damage to the nerve or nerve root that allows elevation of the foot, so that the toes are off the floor while the heel remains down. Immediately I know three things, as would any thinking physician: 1—She has seen another doctor. "Foot drop" is doctor talk. Patients don't say "foot drop" at the first visit. They say, "My foot slaps", "I stub (or catch) my toe", "I trip on curbs", something from daily life. 2—She was not satisfied with what that doctor told her. Otherwise, why is she coming to see me? 3—The third point not everyone will agree with is that she probably does not have foot drop. Patients have an extraordinary way of being right. So I explored further. "Tell me more," I said. "I drag my leg" she replied. Now "drag" means spastic weakness. Foot drop affects the foot; spastic weakness affects the foot and the hip. In both cases, the leg is too long because the foot cannot be elevated. In foot drop compensation is obtained by over flexing the hip to produce what is called a "steppage gait". In spasticity, the weak hip prevents over flexion so the leg is dragged in a circular fashion—so called circumduction. So her weakness was spastic; she was correct to suspect the original diagnosis, "What else?" I asked. "Well," she said, "it's silly, but it's these bubbles" "What bubbles?" I asked. "Little bubbles that keep bursting here and there" That made the diagnosis, for what she was describing was muscle fasciculations, twitches of small muscle fascicles that were in the process of losing their nerve supply. You might have thought she was describing a sensory disorder but paresthesias are usually described as "ginger ale" or "sparkling water" when they are likened to bubbles—a burst of bubbles as when you open the bottle, not single isolated bubbles. She had amyotrophic lateral sclerosis or motor neuron disease, often called Lou Gerhig's Disease. An unfortunate diagnosis confirmed in this patient by the course of events.

This issue of language comes up over and over and is very hard to teach. The Chief Complaint should be entered in the record in the patient's own words, for the way the patient says it is often as revealing as what is said. The words are the medium for conveying information and as the famous phrase has it "The medium is the message" So, in this era of Nurse Practitioners a woman came to the hospital complaining of unsteadiness on her feet. The nurse entered a Chief Complaint of vertigo. Vertigo means dizziness—usually a labyrinthine disorder—so the doctor prescribed a medication for labyrinthitis. The patient returned the next day and a different nurse entered a Chief Complaint of ataxia, which means trouble walking and is often ascribed to a cerebellar disorder. The patient was admitted and within 24 hours was dead of a brain stem stroke. I do not mean to imply that the outcome would have been different if the Chief Complaint had been entered as "unsteady on my feet". I mean to suggest that the patient's words, not somebody else's interpretation translate into doctors diagnoses. Words must not be changed and must be interpreted with care: squeezing or pressure means cardiac, drunk means cerebellar, fizzy water means paresthesias.

Part of the desire to change the words comes, I suspect, from the desire to be more "scientific"—an attitude especially appealing to young doctors and nurses. For years I have listened to student presentations about (for example) a 42 year old "female" or a 63 year old "male" for male and female are obviously more scientific than "man" and "woman". Just before graduation one year, I told a small group of students I was going to give them a gift. That pleased them although the gift did not. "It's the two words man and woman that I offer you for the rest of your careers." They thought I was strange, but that was nothing new. "This is the craziest interview I have ever had" said one applicant to our training program. He had wanted me to review his CV or hear about his laboratory experiments. I knew they would be exemplary. The fact that he was offering them indicated that. I wanted to know could he get out of bed in the morning. The way we train our medical students and young doctors emphasizes the wrong values. Do they know facts which can be tested on written examinations, most of which can be found in reference books, can be learned along the way and will be outdated in many cases by time they come to be used. Better to teach principles, logic, attitudes, and behavior. One young resident whom I had chided asked how I would do it were I in charge. I told her if I had to give ten lectures in Neurology, I would spend five on logic, four on good manners and one on how to use a library. Good manners? you ask. One of the major impediments to learning and caring for patients is a consequence of the competitiveness of the educational system and the aggressiveness it rewards; aggressiveness, which could at least be masked by good manners. Coupled with lack of discipline in our postgraduate training programs it takes a number of years of practice in the real world to burnish the rough edges. One staff member, complaining about the arrogant, ill-mannered behavior of the residents said, "They behave just the way I did when I was a resident" and he was correct, for I remembered his years on the House Staff. Maturity cannot be taught. The paradox is that society picks the best from secondary schools to go to college. The medical schools pick the best college graduates to go to medical school. The hospitals pick the best medical graduates for their training programs and often end up with knowledgeable, aggressive, self centered, immature youngsters with a sense of entitlement, little sense of responsibility and unwillingness to be disciplined. So, I am told at morning report "This 83 year old gomer was admitted because of . . ." One of the definitions of gomer in my dictionary (short for gomeral) is simpleton or fool. "Wait a minute" I interrupt, "This gomer may be somebody's father. He may have had a distinguished career. Even if not he is entitled to your respect." The ethics of equality demand, *"that even the most diminished among us is not denied the respect and care that all human beings are owed"* (The President's Council on Bioethics Washington DC 2005 p.106). Fat chance. I remember the first day in gross anatomy lab when I entered medical school. The professor pointed out, gently but firmly, that these cadavers had been human beings and he would tolerate no disrespect. He established the tone that prevailed in the lab for the entire year. There were no jokes—but that was when students obeyed.

Discipline early in training ingrains attitudes and behavior patterns that persist throughout one's career. The problem is they cannot be taught. They are transmitted by example and in medical training the major exemplar is the doctor a year ahead. Most learning comes from your resident. I interned in a cottage hospital, built on a horizontal plan, and so there was a long trek from House Officers quarters at one end to the wards at the other. Quite late one night the nurse called to tell me Mrs. Soanso needed a laxative.

Telephone orders were not allowed. I got up, got dressed, walked the length of the hospital, entered the ward nursing station, and found my resident there. He could have written the order but he felt it was his job to see if I would come. Had he written the order the laxative would have been just as good. But what he was doing was teaching; something that could not be taught by words.

I still remember that episode, more than 50 years later. And I remember other items from early training because of the discipline that was imposed. We were expected to know our patients in detail, including laboratory results. When the professor asked for the results of the spinal tap and was told it was normal, he said, with some asperity "Just tell me the numbers. I'll decide if it was normal." On presentation of a case, notes were not permitted. Some might consider this unduly severe. Today's House Staff certainly would. But as a result, I have retained a lot of useful information. If you inquired about the level of spinal fluid protein in hypertensive encephalopathy—that is, is the diagnosis excluded by a high level—I know the answer from experience, from a specific patient I recall. As a trainee, I attended out patient clinic (as an observer) at The National Hospital in London. Sir Charles Symonds, recently retired, still appeared on rare occasion as the physician in charge. He was a wise and gracious gentleman. One day he saw a complicated case no one could diagnose. At the end of the examination, after the patient had left he said, "I have seen this once before—about 30 years ago" and then gave a splendid discussion based on his recalled experience. That sort of performance is the product of knowing one's patients in detail without having to refer to notes.

That outpatient experience took place in a small amphitheatre in which the rows of seats rose steeply, so all attendees were visible. One day, after a patient had been presented and had left Sir Charles looked around and said, "Well, what do you think?" His eye fell on me. I looked elsewhere hoping he would too, but when I turned back, his gaze was still on me. I was trapped. I gave him my formulation of the problem and my diagnosis. He pulled his chin silently for a long moment, then said: "I understand your argument but I think my argument is stronger". He then presented his argument; it was stronger. In all my training to that point, I had never been treated like that. He considered what I had to say as if I were an equal. How different from the States where ego was paramount and the "gotcha" approach prevailed, teaching young trainees to be defensive and aggressive.

These teaching conferences were not without their amusing aspects as I discovered later as a teacher. I remember a number of them in which I or another senior faculty member had been asked to analyze a case. The history would be presented, the patient examined then allowed to leave, and the discussant would develop his ideas without advance preparation. It showed the attendees how a senior physician analyzed a problem. It always seemed to me the accuracy of diagnosis was of less importance—after all, the patient had a treating physician—than the method of analysis. Often the best teaching was the result of the worst mistake. Your colleagues and trainees would never forget. Furthermore, they might never let you forget. At one weekly conference, I was shown a man who had decided to get rid of his in—ground swimming pool. One week end he rented a pneumatic hammer and began to break up the concrete. In midmorning, he stopped for coffee. In the kitchen, his hand holding the cup began to shake, spilling the coffee. He thought this was an after effect of the pneumatic hammer but it occurred again later in the day and shortly enough it was evident he was having focal seizures—which indicate a brain lesion. At conference, I discussed all the causes of focal seizures. For years, I had been teaching that one cause always to consider was subacute bacterial endocarditis. Endocarditis is a bacterial infection of the heart valves. Infected clots form on the valve and then may be broken off and thrown to the brain. Endocarditis is a treatable and often curable disease. Guess what I forgot to mention at that conference. In the subsequent days, more clots were thrown to the brain, and the patient had two strokes with paralysis. At the next week's conference the first thing I did, as always, was ask for a follow up on the previous week's patient. I was told he had subacute bacterial endocarditis and had had two strokes. I said that was my fault, that I had neglected to suggest the correct diagnosis and that this patient's bad outcome was the result of my oversight. I emphasized the point, for I felt it was bad that I had overlooked the diagnosis but that at least I should try to salvage the teaching point. Emphasizing my mistake would help the group remember for life that "Locke missed it" and that they must not make the same mistake. From the back of the room came the voice of a senior member of the Infectious Disease group. "Dr. Locke" he said, "that was an impossible diagnosis to make. You should not be so hard on yourself. Nobody could have made the correct diagnosis until the patient had his stroke." "What are you doing?" I thought to myself. "Don't you understand I am teaching?" If no one could do it, we are all excused. If no one is to blame it will be OK to miss it the next time" But of course these were not points to be made out loud. This approach—and I understand my colleague was being a gentleman—reflects our current concern with self-esteem and our unwillingness to accept responsibility, to be real doctors.

If no one is to blame who is responsible for this patient's care and for the bad outcome? By accepting blame, by accepting responsibility, perhaps I can serve as a so-called role model for my young colleagues. To have this undermined by a gracious staff member only perpetuates the unwillingness of the young doctor to be responsible.

At one such conference I discussed a difficult case in detail, localized the lesion with precision, chose from a list of possible causes, and talked about treatment and the outlook for recovery. At the conclusion of the conference, a student came up. "That was a great discussion," he said. "We thought this was a very interesting case so we presented it to Dr. Watsisname who was visiting from New York". "What did he think?" I asked. "Oh" said the student "he didn't know either". Who says teaching is without rewards.

More rewarding was the young black student who talked with me after a conference on aphasia—a disorder of language resulting from a brain lesion. My ideas on aphasia were out of the main stream of that period and the black student was in medical school at a time there were few blacks there. "That was very exciting", he said. "Your ideas raise a lot of interesting issues for me to think about. But, you know" he said "for the moment I've got one job and one job only, and that's to get out of medical school, so I'm going to have to tell it to them their way". A summary statement about the conformation we impose in medical school on the creative or original thinker

Another interesting interaction occurred with a minority student. Faculty members would meet once a week with four senior students. One week two of my students were off on internship interviews, a third was sick, so the remaining student, a Hispanic, and I were alone. As a result, the conversation became more intimate than usual. He told me he had found medical school hard. As a member of a minority he was not understood, he was not prepared, expectations of him were too high and anyhow he was only planning to go back to the *barrio* to take care of his own people; he didn't need to know all the high level medicine used to treat the Boston upper class. "Look at it from my point of view" I said. "My job is to train good doctors no matter where they practice. So I'm going to kick your ass until you become the best God damned doctor you can possibly be and bring the best medicine you can to the *barrio*". He was outraged, but shortly enough his rotation on our service ended and I did not see him again. However, two things happened that may not be related. First, in June, just before graduation, I got a letter from him saying he had thought about what I had said. I was right, and he thanked me. A short time later, I got a letter from the Dean saying that my name was to be included on the short list of candidates for Best Teacher of the year. I did not get the award, but have always supposed my Hispanic student proposed me. And I hadn't even taught him facts.

One of the most amusing conferences took place when a resident on my service discovered a previously undiagnosed case of general paresis. GP, as it is called, is late stage syphilis, and is rarely seen now a days. It is manifest by dementia and a characteristic dysarthria among other things. The old timers could recognize it by the patient's speech and one of my experienced teachers used to say "Don't tell me the Wasserman"—a blood test for syphilis—"just let me hear the patient say 'baby hippopotamus'". I had not seen enough tertiary syphilis to appreciate the typical speech nor had most doctors of my generation. In the front of the auditorium, the Professor was examining the patient. It was clear she had dementia. What was not clear to him was the cause—and he was a specialist in dementia. He struggled to strike on the etiology. Now, for this story to make sense you need to know that our hospital had an ambulatory unit where diabetic patients came to learn about management of their disease: food values, insulin doses, and things of that sort in lectures given by diabetologists in various amphitheatres in the hospital. These patients were issued red vinyl covered three ring loose leaf binders with outlines of the lectures they attended, and they could be seen in the hospital corridors carrying their red loose leaf books on the way to lectures. While the professor struggled to determine a diagnosis the door to the auditorium opened, a little old man carrying the tell tale red binder shuffled in, and looked around as the door closed behind him. He spotted the empty seat the Professor had vacated next to me in the first row and came over. It was clear he was in the wrong auditorium, and I gave him some minutes to discover this while I attempted to formulate a graceful way to tell him, should he not leave on his own. He watched the proceedings with interest while the Professor continued to strive for a diagnosis. Unexpectedly he poked me in the ribs with his elbow, leaned over and whispered "She's got syphilis". "How do you know?" I asked. "I've practiced in Brooklyn for forty years" he said. "I see it all the time". Some time later I told this to the Professor; he didn't think it was funny.

Doctor's egos often get in the way like that. At one conference at which I was a member of the audience, a young man with an unusual brain stem lesion was presented. Among other conditions was the possibility this was infectious. I suggested, when the discussion was opened to the audience, this might be caused by a rare organism called Petrolidium boydii. This did not attract much attention because the organism was not known by most. Only about twenty cases had appeared in the world literature. However, one of the residents carried my suggestion to Chief's report at which the entire resident staff met with the Chief of Medicine once a week. The Chief was an expert in infectious disease; in fact, he once was President of the Infectious Disease Society of America. What I know is by hearsay only, but I was told he rejected my suggestion as unreasonable. The patient lingered for many weeks, then ultimately came to postmortem examination at which he was found to be infected by the organism I had suggested. I had a congratulatory note from one of the younger members of the Infectious Disease Section. The Chief of Medicine said nothing. A short time later I was relieved of my position (which I served at the pleasure of the Chief of Medicine) as Chief of the Neurology Section.

It has always seemed to me that in these teaching conferences, as in diagnosis of a patient in a clinical setting, all available information, medical and otherwise, was to be used. So, when I was once presented with a difficult case (later to be published) and told at the outset that this still undiagnosed patient had been presented to four colleagues separately, each of whom was named, I felt I could use that information. I knew these doctors; I knew how they thought. There was no point in reiterating diagnoses they, in all probability, had already offered. That narrowed the field considerably and forced me to a correct diagnosis of progressive multifocal leukoencephalopathy, at a time when that was an unfamiliar disorder to most. Do you remember the childhood puzzle of the three red dots? A rich man tells his three sons he will place a red dot or a black dot on the forehead of each of his blindfolded boys. When the blinds are removed they are to raise a hand if they see a red dot. The first boy to figure out the color of the dot on his forehead inherits the father's fortune. He then places a red dot on each forehead, unblinds the boys and watches as three hands go up. There is a long pause, then one boy (he would be the youngest in a proper fairy tale) says "I know, I've got a red spot". How did he know? The answer is that he knew his brothers just as I knew my colleagues. Had there been two red dots three hands would have been raised. "My brother, seeing three hands and my black dot would have said he had a red dot. But he didn't say anything. Therefore I must have a red dot."

All too often doctors need to do something. Their egos require it, their patients demand it, insurance companies reimburse it. Often it is exactly wrong. We do too much. We kill with overtreatment. One recent study found that patients managed by critical care physicians had a 47% higher risk of death than patients managed by non-critical care physicians in the Intensive Care Unit. Exactly the reverse of what you might guess—perhaps because the critical care doctors do too much (Levy, M. Ann Int Med, June 3, 2008). One of the best doctors I knew would say to anyone who would listen "Remember, sometimes doing nothing is doing something." But I was one of the few willing to listen. We have a mind set. Part of it comes from training. Part of it comes with our specialty. If you are an emergency room physician everything is an emergency. An orthopedist sent me a young woman who was having trouble walking, after he had operated on her knee. Her trouble walking was caused by multiple sclerosis. Shouldn't I have seen her before he did something?

We saw a patient in Intensive Care, admitted for a heart attack. I no longer remember why we saw him but it was not for the droopy eyelid I noticed but did not record in my note. In the corridor when I discussed the findings with the residents and the fourth year medical student I said "I suspect you saw the droopy eyelid and recognized it as a manifestation of ocular myasthenia" Ocular myasthenia is a benign disorder of the elderly, often best left alone. Aggressive treatment in a man who has just had a heart attack could be dangerous. "But you didn't say anything about it in your note" said the student. "Of course not" I said "I don't want them treating him". "But that's malpractice" said the student. "I should report you" Fortunately he didn't, but it shows the mind set of the young with respect to "doing something".

Often the ascription of success is to having done something. I had a patient with metastatic cancer of the breast. Her primary lesion had been surgically treated when, some time later, she showed up with a brain tumor. The brain tumor was a distant spread of the breast cancer. Discussion with the patient and her husband elicited the request to "do everything possible". In due course, a neurosurgeon removed the brain tumor, a general surgeon removed her adrenals, an oncologist treated her with chemotherapy, a radiologist provided x-ray therapy to the brain at the end of which her husband told me he had just read an advertisement for an excursion trip to Lourdes and asked if he could take his wife. I said certainly if she felt able to make the trip. I ran into her two years later in the Chicago airport. She looked like a million bucks—as if she had just stepped out of a bandbox. As you might expect the neurosurgeon felt he had been responsible for the cure, the general surgeon thought it was the removal of the adrenals, the oncologist attributed it to the chemotherapy, the radiologist to the effects of the x-ray therapy and the patient and her husband thought it was the result of the pilgrimage to Lourdes. Decision about this sort of aggressive therapy must rest with the patient and is always a reflection of the individual's personality. An aggressive trial lawyer who had taken the bull by the horns all his life wanted his metastatic brain tumor from lung removed despite my discouraging him, so I acceded to what proved to be a bad outcome.

These kinds of decisions by the physician and by the patient are less frequent now that the insurance companies are in charge. They often decide what constitutes standard of practice and control the situation by reimbursement. This may be determined by physicians employed by the insurance companies, or may be undertaken by outside firms in the pay of the insurance company. They provide so-called "independent medical examinations" at their offices on a fee for service basis to independent physicians. In order to continue in service the opinions of the doctors must in the end be favorable to the insurance companies, In my experience the situation is unacceptable. The "independent" companies are usually run, if not owned, by former insurance adjusters. They read each report and often "adjust" it. I would be asked to sign reports different from what I had dictated. On occasion, I would find my signature (without initials) on reports I had never signed. I refused to provide a rubber stamp signature they could use to "speed up turn around time"

Even direct reimbursement has problems. Never mind the level of payment, which may or may not be adequate. A typical example, using Medicare as representative, is for an internist to charge $149 for an initial one-hour consultation. Medicare approves $71.41 and pays 80% of the approved amount or $57.13. A Ford dealership labor charge (in the same geographic area) is $89.00 an hour—$31.87 more than is paid the internist or 155% of what the doctor gets. At one time Blue Cross Blue Shield of Massachusetts paid a specified amount for a hospital consultation and nothing for the first four follow up visits. Only with the fifth hospital visit was additional reimbursement provided. Discussing this with a Blue Cross representative I asked what was the impetus for a doctor to follow a hospital patient and was told "good practice". I do not know whether this custom still persists.

Some doctors have had good success refusing insurance. The patient pays the doctor's fee and is reimbursed at the insurance company's rate. This has worked well for a group of neurologists in Salt Lake City and for an internist (loosely affiliated with similar internists to allow cross coverage) in Pasadena. A hybrid approach has recently appeared in the formation of "concierge doctors". Begun in 1996 there about 5000 doctors not intimately related to hospital departments who accept insurance and the mandated rates, but have a group of "preferred patients" who get preferential and rapid entry into the system—which is why, I suspect, these doctors are termed "concierge", for like the Parisian door keeper they control entry. As a patient, you can join such a practice for an annual fee that ranges from about $1500 to as much as $25000 depending on the doctor and the size of the practice. Membership offers some degree of immediate attention. Doctors in a concierge program (also called boutique medicine, retainer medicine, platinum practice, executive health program, personalized health care, luxury health care, and fee for non-covered service) have a practice of the order of 300-600 patients in contrast to the roughly 3000 necessary in a regular insurance covered program. Most accept insurance so as not to violate contract obligations, in addition to the concierge retainer which is specified to cover non insured services including rapid access (same or next day), longer visits, Saturday appointments, 24 hour telephone response, house calls, check ups and some other services not covered by insurance, such as arranged hospital admissions or visits to specialists. One might anticipate this kind of program would favor wealthy patients but experience reveals that fewer rich patients contracted for concierge care than did middle class. The reason?: the rich are often socially prominent, are hospital donors, have political connections. They do not need a concierge program to get special care. While offering more personalized care, reminiscent of the bygone individual fee for service era, the retainer contract must not promise more or better diagnostic or therapeutic services; the American Medical Association ethical guidelines mandate equal quality of care for patients paying extra and those who are not. The bygone fee for service era is also recalled by the inclusion of indigent patients in programs such as the one in Palm Beach County where concierge physicians who donate several hours a month offer free doctor care to uninsured patients. As of July 2008, about 400 Palm Beach County physicians were participating. "Scholarship patients" are estimated to constitute 10% of the roster. This program is implemented by MDVIP the company that runs the largest concierge practice in the country. It screens and selects physicians, provides services it considers critical for a successful practice and receives a portion of the annual membership fee. It has established a "Medical Centers of Excellence" program that provides members access to "premiere academic institutions in the nation". There VIP service is offered: appointments are facilitated, transfer of medical records arranged, help is provided with travel plans and guiding the patient through the facility is offered. But cost of medical services is the patient's responsibility. MDVIP ambiguously reports that "patients are admitted to the hospital at dramatically lower rates"—up to 65% for Medicare patients and up to 80% for patients covered by commercial insurance; what is not clear is whether rate means financial (daily charges) or frequency of admission. Does it mean the result of their preventive care programs, shorter stays, less severe illness or reduced charges to their patients?

For the physician the concierge concept offers longer time with the patient, a smaller patient load, and a good financial return. Instead of 25-35 patients a day with appointments limited to 15 or 20 minutes (resulting in a ten or twelve hour day when chart notes, telephone time and other incidentals are included), a primary care physician whose retainer is $1000 can anticipate an annual income of $300,000 in addition to insurance income with a roster of 300 patients; 10% of the number of patients needed under an entirely insurance financed program. The insurance income can now be used exclusively for overhead: rent, telephone, secretary, nurse—a not inconsiderable part of a practitioner's gross income. The problem with this approach is that it restores the old inequality of medical care according to financial criteria despite the small number of scholarship patients. It is an obvious indicator that the current system is inadequate, at least according to the criteria of the middle class.

At the financial interface of the hospital and the hospital doctors (other than House Staff) is the Professional Organization. This usually consists of all staff doctors of a given hospital department, grouped under the rubric of a professional organization for billing purposes. Outside doctors or members of another hospital in the consortium may belong. Insurance reimbursement characteristically comes in two categories: one for hospital services and one for professional services. The hospital may be paid for the performance of a test or for the office space used by the doctor in the hospital. The doctor may be paid for the interpretation of a test or for the examination in the hospital office space. Billing takes place in several steps, some of which are performed by hospital employees, some by the Professional Organization. Members of the Professional Organization usually have little idea of what is being billed. They are usually reimbursed a fixed annual amount by the department (adjusted periodically) which they are expected to generate from clinical practice. Their revenue contributes to departmental expenses such as secretaries who have no commitment to a given doctor and, while interposed between patient and doctor, have neither interest in nor knowledge of the patient. Although it is never expressed this way, these departmental doctors, while technically not hospital employees, are effectively working for the hospital. So the old tripartite dynamic division of hospital, doctor and patient has given way to the distinction (and opposition) employed by the insurance companies of provider and consumer, an adversary relationship like that of buyer and seller with the hospital and doctor combined in the role of provider.

A Professional Organization may provide service to more than 1500 members. It assumes responsibility for benefits management, payroll, financial and accounting services, business development and analysis, oversight and training. It includes physicians, podiatrists, and psychologists. An annual budget may be 250 million dollars, one fifth of which may come from the hospital as reimbursement for physician administrative duties, medical education and hospital billed patient services. Each department is expected to submit a break even annual budget. Department heads sit on the Board of Managers of the Professional Organization. Notice that it is a hospital department, the physicians of which generate the major income for the Professional Organization, that relates to the organization so that, once again, the distinction between doctor and hospital is eroded. The hospital's goals rather than patient needs become the doctor's goals. Nonetheless, the Professional Organization continues to advertise a mission "to promote . . . the best quality and value of care to patients". (Website BIDPO 6/30/08) Only the term value reveals the dominant role of money as a consideration. Like the physician pod, the Professional Organization can be structured to accept risk-based managed care contracts that serve as further incentive for monetary considerations to become paramount in decisions about patient care. It determines contract terms, criteria, policies, fee schedules, and division of revenues and is responsible for medical management. Medical management enables physicians to improve the efficiency of care by addressing such things as utilization, cost, and quality that will produce the best outcome for patient care but also for contract performance. Financially integrated contracts, which are incentive and risk based are available for professional organizations as well as for independent physician groups and puts the physician in the role of a stockholder in a corporation—if the company makes money the stockholder makes money, if the corporation takes a loss so does the stockholder (or the physician), Committees review and advise on prescription of medication insuring compliance with the approved formulary and analyze and review out of network referrals thereby limiting the independent judgement of an individual physician. These committees may "assist physicians in understanding and achieving our Pay for Performance incentives administered by various payers" (Medical Management 3/24/08)

Most doctors can't be bothered with all of this. They want to take care of their patients and seek the easiest way. They don't know (and don't want to know) the details of the financial aspects. They are ready to do as they are told so long as it does not fly in the face of good care. They are paid regularly, usually at an agreed rate determined in part by academic level. They sign a contract with the Professional Organization and accept what they are paid without understanding the details. The individual program may include a bonus provision so that guaranteed reimbursement is based on an anticipated number of patients and is provided whether that number is achieved or not. If that number is exceeded the physician may receive up to 50% of the excess reimbursement, the additional 50% being distributed to the department. The patient, like the doctor, is usually excluded from the financial details, and like the doctor usually does not care just as long as payment is taken care of. The patient has no financial obligation to the doctor, need not be satisfied with the relationship for the doctor to be paid and the doctor, in turn, is absolved of any financial incentive to have a personal relationship with the patient. The doctor's relationship is now with the insurance carrier. Patient satisfaction has given way to insurance company satisfaction, and this creates a paradox. Just as the doctor-patient, relationship is adversarial, so too the doctor-insurance company interaction is adversarial.

A major shift in the culture of the medical community occurred with the rise of feminism in society. Several waves of attack, motivated by a changing ideology, occurred in a period of years, the result of which is that now it is not infrequent for a medical school class to have more women than men. One might have anticipated a return to some of the older values of patient care in light of the argument that women are more compassionate than men are, but this has not happened. What has happened is that some concessions to motherhood have been required, family values have intruded on medical training and the physical demands, such as hours on duty, have been reduced. Still, one hears talk about inequities and unfairness. All of which brings to mind my Aunt Sophie, who graduated medical school in 1921, and maintained a busy and socially useful practice caring for a large population of indigents. She married, raised a son who recently retired from medical practice, without interrupting her practice, without whining or talking about glass ceilings. She practiced for over 40 years and then retired. But retirement was unsatisfying so she joined Volunteers in Service to America (VISTA), and did two tours of duty in Appalachia. For her third reenlistment, she was sent to California, where before long she was called before the Board of Registration in Medicine for writing prescriptions without a California license. She explained she was working for the Federal government but was told that did not matter; she was still required to have a California license. "What do

I have to have to do to obtain a California license?" she asked and was told she must take an oral examination. So, well over the age of 70, she appeared before the Board to be examined by "Three nice boys" she said. They must have been over the age of 50. They asked a number of medical questions, then, one presented a hypothetical case of a man with a fever and pulmonary findings. "What would you think of?" he asked. Sophie thought for a moment, then said, "Well I suppose I'd have to consider coccidioidomycosis". That disorder is almost specific to the San Fernando Valley in California and not familiar to most physicians outside the area. "If you know that," said the examiner "I guess we'll have to give you your license". So, Sophie continued her good work for several more years, unimpeded.

One of the demands of the feminists was to remove paternalism from the practice of medicine, a demand the profession acceded to more than two decades ago. A noble impulse that perhaps overlooks the role of magical thinking on the parts of many patients (more about that later). The patient with incurable cancer puts faith in the power of the doctor to help, if not to cure. Remnants of the "Daddy, fix" attitude left over from childhood are present in many of us. That attitude by the patient, unrealistic though it be, may serve as a powerful tool in the care of the patient, although it may be useless in the cure of the patient. The well-known placebo effect is not really an effect of the placebo. It is the effect of a placebo administered by the doctor. It is an effect of the doctor-patient relationship, of the patient's trust in the doctor and it raises problems for the ethicist (see Emanuel, E. in the British Medical Journal October 23, 2008) who notes the paradox of treating the patient with a placebo about which the patient is unaware, and the stated policy that the patient must be an enlightened participant in all decisions. But you can't have it both ways. A surprisingly large number of physicians prescribe placebos without disclosing their use, for disclosure would defeat the purpose. The most common description to the patient is a "potentially beneficial medicine". The unrealistic ethicist might confront the dilemma by suggesting the physician waffle with some such statement as "I'm not sure this drug will work", a statement that at the outset undermines the effect of the placebo—a self-fulfilling prophesy. How does one deal with children? Do you always tell the unvarnished truth and have them participate in all decisions? If part of the sick, anxious, frightened patient is a reflection of, a regression to, childhood behavior patterns, perhaps the academic adult oriented ethicist should not partake.

The transfer in attitude from patient care to patient treatment (if not cure) is perhaps most sharply demonstrated in psychiatry in the movement away from psychotherapy with it's intense relationship between doctor and patient, to psychopharmacology where the pill can be prescribed with only an occasional visit to the doctor. Which is better? Each supplies something the other does not. Perhaps they should be employed in concert. However, that would not be the most efficient, most economical way. Medicine may not be a cottage industry but it should not be an industry at all. Efficiency and economy should not be criteria of good care. If the practice of medicine is an art, as we once believed, (Hippocrates said, "Life is short and the art long") it cannot be efficient. Unless it be an art in which you paint by the numbers.

PATIENTS

Patients are harder to discuss than are doctors or hospitals, for patients are individuals. Doctors and hospitals are individual too, but they have group characteristics, behavior, and motives. It is harder to define group behavior or desires for patient populations although certain characteristics may unify them. The most unifying is that all patients come for help. They are, to use an old-fashioned word, suppliants. In response, the temptation for the doctor is to be imperious, authoritative, commanding. The stage is set for an unbalanced relationship because of the position from which each arrives. The relation is unbalanced in reality with respect to the knowledge or expertise the doctor brings to the engagement; that is why the patient comes. But that position of authority with respect to knowledge must also bring with it humility. The patient must always be respected as an integral individual independent of the disease it bears. Supplication comes in a variety of forms, some of which obscure the real meaning. Patients may be demanding, may appear unconcerned, may be noncompliant, argumentative, or offensively hostile but they are all there to ask for help. Otherwise, why did they come? It is easy for the doctor to lose sight of that, to be put off by the façade, but recognition of the cause of the visit—the call for help—keeps the relationship where it belongs. All patients want restoration of health, all want comfort, and want to be free of pain. However, what constitutes pain for one may not be pain for another, the degree of acceptable discomfort may vary, and attitudes and emotions may be unknowns or imponderables that enter into a patient's behavior. Obviously, the best understanding of a patient comes from a longitudinal relationship. The old family doctor excelled at this; current organization precludes it. A cartoon shows the doctor entering the waiting room from the office and saying to the assembled patients "My name is David. I'll be your doctor today". Like so much of humor, it is based on truth.

Of course, the doctor—patient relationship depends on what the patient brings to it just as much as it does on what the doctor brings to it. The change of doctor-patient interaction reflects a change that has occurred in many aspects of society. *Caveat emptor* has moved into medicine; after all, the patient is now a consumer, a buyer. The problem is that this adversary attitude undermines an important aspect of the therapeutic relationship. No one helps any longer, so why should the doctor. The shop girl of old (who has become a sales lady then an associate) who said "That looks very good on you Madam", the friendly local grocer of Norman Rockwell Americana no longer exist. Big box stores offer a product only, in an impersonal way. And now, some offer retail clinics, staffed by Nurse Practitioners who provide "off the rack" medicine for $59 a visit. This may reflect the fact that a new patient appointment with a primary care physician may take as long as 100 days in Massachusetts with an average wait of almost two months. This has not increased significantly during the last four years despite the recent advent of mandatory health insurance, for up to 27% of the newly mandated insured population—the lowest economic group—continues to use Emergency Rooms as the initial facility

The long wait for an appointment has prompted a new approach in which patients are seen more promptly, do not feel rushed, and get to spend 90 minutes with the doctor. The doctor, in this program sees more patients in the same period, gets more money, though charging the same fee, and does not have to repeat the same instructions several times a day. This is done by having several (up to 8 or 10) patients with the same disorder (cardiac problems, for example) examined in a group. Usually they are not disrobed; if they must be, they are taken out of the group for examination. Otherwise, all members of the group are examined together, treated together, and instructed together. Patients have the option of whether to enter such a program, and 77% of those who do, like it. And we worry about doctor—patient relationships.

So, "Can I trust my doctor? I'd better keep an eye on him". I open the door to the waiting room to introduce myself to the next new patient. He is joined as I invite him in by a young woman. "Who is this?" I ask him, for he is my patient, not the young woman. "I am a patient advocate" she replies as she picks up her pencil and stenographic pad. "I thought that was my job," I say. He indicates he wants her present. She joins us but does not take many notes. Patients in this adversary atmosphere contribute to Angie's List that evaluates "plumbers, painters, movers, and now doctors". Your doctor is positioned with other tradesmen.

Part of the lack of trust may be a problem of communication by the doctor and the problem of communication represents, in part, a lack of time. However, it also represents the difficulty of communicating, impartially, complex medical concepts, and the problem of dealing with patient preconceptions generated by "How To Books", the internet, and Drug Company advertising. The patient who confronts the doctor with a demand for an inappropriate medication creates a difficult decision: either comply or send the patient elsewhere. The old distinction between patient needs and patient wants persists and is difficult to "communicate" in an atmosphere of patient distrust.

What can I do to indicate I am on my patient's side? Most of my colleagues were on the patient's side. I met the Chief of Surgery coming into the hospital one Saturday night at about 11 PM just as I was leaving. "What are you doing here at this hour?" I asked. "It's such a privilege," he said. "I was called away from a dinner party to help with a case." A privilege; a dinner party. And he meant it. He was on his patient's side.

Why bother to know the patient? What difference does it make? After all, the drug is the same whether the patient is known or not. Perhaps some patients do not want the treatment—let's say chemotherapy. Should the doctor insist? Is the decision unilateral? An older colleague pointed out to me gently, when I was a young practitioner that because a treatment is right (I think he meant scientifically) does not mean it is good (I think he meant morally). The patient must participate however irrational the patient's choice might seem, for the choice deals with the patient's body. But it also deals with that irrational thing called mind. Attitudes, beliefs, feelings, and fears enter into the decision. I remember a psychiatrist, many years ago, was asked to see a dying man who was angry at his impending death. The nurses thought it would be better were he to die peacefully. The psychiatrist spent some time with the patient, then said: "He's been an angry man all his life. That's his style. Let's not try to change him now." The invoking of style recalls the old aphorism: "If you're playing a game, the outcome of which is a foregone conclusion, the only thing that matters is the style with which you play". If you are going to die anyway, you might as well do it with style, and it helps if your doctor understands your style.

And the style of your family, for they are also part of your illness, even if it is not terminal. The wife of a dermatological patient spoke of "our skin disease" so even if not a caretaker, (who has no other life) in the sense of the spouse of a patient with Alzheimer's disease, the illness is shared. Just as patient's attitudes vary, so family attitudes vary. I was asked to see a world famous organist in his terminal illness. As I entered his room on the Emergency Ward, the first vision was of a pair of very large hands—farmer's hands—hanging over the side of the gurney. The next sight was of his wife sitting quietly alongside. He died moments later, before I could be of any help. His wife, sensing his departure, said, "I have so much to be grateful for. We had a wonderful life together"

Contrast that with the wife of a man who was brought to the hospital because of a major heart attack. "How could he do that to me?" she complained. "He knew we had tickets to Bermuda". A self-centered remark but also, I suspect, a way of verbalizing the disruption of her life (in the much larger sense than Bermuda, for she might lose her husband), and her grief. Now to try to rally her for his illness is really her illness too; he will need her help physically and emotionally in the long recovery process. How to rally her? "I know it's hard on you" I say "but it's also hard on him. He's going to need you, so you must be strong". Will it work? I don't l know because I don't know her. She is not my patient (neither was he; I was seeing him for a potential neurological complication). I have no relationship with her, nothing I can call on to help her.

People are different. An old Jewish man sat just outside the door of his wife's room as he had for days. She was comatose and the likelihood of her regaining consciousness was minimal. He looked exhausted. I stopped to talk with him as I did each day after my visit to his wife. "Why don't you go home and get some rest?" I advised. "She doesn't know you are here". "Dr. Locke he replied, "I have been married to this woman for 47 years. There are principles." Principles! I felt about two inches tall. People do not talk about principles anymore. This man summarized—in a different context—what is wrong with the doctor-patient relationship now a days. And I fear there is no going back. Not only do we not try to teach our students medical principles, only facts, neither do we try to teach them moral or ethical principles. In any case it is probably too late. This teaching has to begin at home, by example and at an early age. A violinist from the Symphony came to see me. During our conversation, I asked him if he had started to study the violin at an early age. "No" he said "I was five". Ethical principles, like the violin, must be learned when very young.

Patient and family involvement in decisions about treatment is an ethical notion that is loaded with difficulties. It does not distinguish scientific fact, about which there can be little dispute, from values, moral judgements, attitudes, beliefs, prejudices and all other things (sugar and spice) humans are made of. The facts change with time, which is why medical certainty must be tempered with judgement, but at a given moment they are the best we have and should be used. Periodically, when meeting with students, I would be told by one of them that something I had said was not right. "How many of you think he is right?" my adversary would ask the other students. Each time I would have to explain that I am a strong proponent of participatory democracy but there are certain things that cannot be put to a vote. "Let's look it up" I would suggest. However, whatever the fact, it, by itself, cannot determine the therapeutic decision

In this era of equality it is, perhaps, not surprising that young doctors behave as they do. Radio news broadcasts are populated by the "man on the street". Bloggers offer an endless supply of opinions about anything you want. Encyclopedias are fashioned out of common knowledge. Experts are considered "elite"—a pejorative. One opinion is as good as another, and we collect them as if we were anthropologists. Yet, I remember one professor of anthropology who during the era when students demanded "relevance" said that for years she had resisted the University administration's efforts to tell her what to teach; she was not now prepared to have the students tell her what to teach. Indeed, the whole notion of teacher and student presupposes that one knows more than the other—that the relation is asymmetric. This is perhaps most true in the hard sciences. Facts change, but at any given period they are immutable, or at least indisputable, until revised. They serve as the basis for behavior. They can be taught. There are experts. One opinion is not as good as another; this should fashion the relation between trainee and supervisor and between doctor and patient. The topic of patient participation has been captured by bioethicists, often theorists, not caretakers, who view the problem in an abstract way. Far different from the problems faced by the treating physician and the patient in the real world. Part of the difficulty relates to the inability of the abstract discussion to take into consideration the large variety of factors—other than intellectual—that influence patient's decisions. Emotions, beliefs, attitudes, finances, and a host of other imponderables are known to the patient's physician but not to the ethicists who are not caring for them. "I have enough money to be well" said one man with a job and with life insurance but with no health insurance "and enough money to be dead, but not enough money to be sick". Will that influence his decisions? Will that influence the ethicist's decisions? Will the ethicist even know? Even well meaning doctors, who talk of "empowering" (again the arrogance—the doctor gives the power) the patient to participate in the decision overlook the subtleties involved. Worse, they overlook their roles in the presentation of data—not without a point of view. What is offered is not a neutral commodity; it is a biased statement. And it is freighted with the relationship. Remember the days of the "good patient"? A good patient does what the doctor suggests. Will the patient who does not follow advice destroy the relationship? Does that possibility enter into the patient's mind and into the decision? All too often, the physician, like the ethicist, sees the decision as an academic problem with a right or wrong dichotomy, rather than the nuanced, complicated phenomenon it really is. Because of this patients are better qualified to make judgements about what they do not want—negative judgements—than about what they do want—positive decisions. It is proper for a patient to reject a procedure or a course of action for reasons that are not evident, not expressed, or even not rational. It may not be proper for a patient to choose a course of action for reasons that are not evident or not rational. Every course of action is presented by a partisan. Isn't that the reason for a second opinion. A woman went to a surgeon when she found a lump in her remaining breast. Surgery was recommended. What did she expect? The doctor was a surgeon. "At least I'll be symmetrical," she said. There is no way, despite the best intentions, for the doctor to present all the information that must enter into the patient's decision in an unbiased, dispassionate way, and no way for the ethicist (and sometimes even the caregiver) to understand all the factors that enter into the patient's decision. Furthermore, making the patient a participant in the decision absolves the doctor of responsibility of an unfavorable outcome. After all, it was the patient who chose. The President's Council on Bioethics writes in September 2005 (pages 157-158) "In reality, individuals, though free to choose, never simply decide solely by and for themselves, even when they are fully competent. The present patient's decisions reflect, in part, his image of himself in the eyes of others, and his decisions affect the course of their lives. More generally, our identity and values always take shape within a network of human relations. The individual may know himself from the inside, but his inside knowledge is shaped by his understanding of how others understand him. And his inside knowledge, never final or definitive, is always open to transformations of self-understanding in light of new circumstances, at least as long as he is still self aware. A discussion with those affected by his decision or with his trusted physician could very well lead to such a transformation of outlook". Furthermore, though the individual is "free to choose" (whatever that means) " . . . family members are rarely the only actors in this drama: there are doctors, hospitals, and nursing homes who make recommendations about best care; there are insurance companies and governments that pay a large fraction of health care and long-term costs for the elderly and that decide what they will pay for; there is the larger polity that must weigh these goods against other civic goods; and there are the fundamental values of society such as nurturing the young, securing the equal rights of all, and protecting the vulnerable from harm. Thus, although individuals may not aim at the good of society in making decisions, society as a whole establishes conditions that powerfully influence and constrain those decisions—including the influence of law and culture on the ethical intuitions of the individuals who bear the responsibility of care." (page 125). Because morality is a communal function " . . . moral intuitions do not develop out of nowhere; they are shaped by the ethos of the society in which we live, by the general culture and specific guidelines that govern the practice of medicine, and by the role models who serve as our teachers and our guides" (page 99). Still, it must be the patient's decision, not the family's, that is to be honored.

Often the patient is not able to decide. Clinical state, medication, uncertainty, preclude participation. If there is not a designated medical surrogate who, if anyone, should take part with the doctor? What if a family is divided on a course of action; the spouse cannot decide and the children have conflicting interests. Often when able to take part, the patient, no matter how intelligent, how well educated, will not, (or cannot) understand the implications of what is being presented. The mode of presentation combined with the hopes of the patient may determine the decision. A New Hampshire town manager was sent to Boston some two weeks after having suffered a subarachnoid hemorrhage. Usually a subarachnoid hemorrhage is from a ruptured aneurysm, a bubble on an artery that represents a weak spot—like a bubble on a garden hose. It may grow in size until one day it bursts, pouring blood all around the brain, but not destroying brain tissue. (When it bleeds into brain, it is called a meningocerebral hemorrhage). The aneurysm may clot, the bleeding stop, and repair occur; or the aneurysm can be treated surgically. The possibility of rebleed declines during the early weeks following the initial bleed, so that by the third week after onset the incidence of rebleed was less than the incidence of surgical complications in the era in which this man was seen. His aneurysm was on the anterior communicating artery, between the frontal lobes and behind the eyes. The only neurological complication he had experienced resulted from the extension of blood along the optic nerves into his retinae, causing some loss of vision, but this would clear as the blood was resorbed from the subhyaloid space. This intelligent man wanted information about his disorder so he could choose a course of action. We talked about the nature of the process, and the medical and surgical options for treatment. He asked me about the medical treatment. Could he rebleed? "Yes" I said. Could the rebleed cause damage to his brain? "Yes" I said. Was rebleed likely? "Unpredictable" I said, "but less and less likely with the passage of each week" Could he see a neurosurgeon?" Yes" I said, and returned some time later with a neurosurgical colleague. "I can cure you," said the surgeon. The patient looked at me, offered his hand for me to shake, and said "Thank you Dr. Locke". I had been dismissed. The choice was easy: one doctor spoke of uncertainty and rebleed, the second spoke of cure. Postoperatively he presented the typical picture of akinetic mutism, a syndrome that may result from damage in the region of the third ventricle or the frontal interhemispheric region. He would stand immobile for long periods at the foot of his bed, though he could move all four limbs, and would not speak. His surgeon felt the procedure had been a success; the aneurysm had been isolated and taken out of the circulation of blood. It would not rebleed. I felt the procedure may have been a surgical success with respect to isolation of the aneurysm but had been a failure from the viewpoint of the patient who would not be able to return to his job, to an independent life and to his community and his family. My colleague was not a mean or uncaring man. He simply had different criteria. However, those criteria were instrumental in the patient's decision. He was told he would be cured, and he was cured of his aneurysm. He didn't think to ask (who would) will I be able to go back to work, will I be able to be a good husband and father, will I be able to have fun. From my point of view, he had made the wrong decision despite my efforts to give him the best information, but all too often, the best information is not the basis on which the patient decides. More often, it is hope, denial, and the human need for magic. For many of us magic is left over from childhood. We do not usually acknowledge it until a crisis, such as illness, appears. Then the doctor is a powerful person, the episode will have a happy ending. This magic was familiar to Sir William Osler who wrote more than a century ago "The desire to take medicine is perhaps the greatest feature which distinguishes man from animals". Sick people, writes the New York Times (August 26, 2008) "wish away their symptoms then move smoothly from denial to deception". If you try to explain to your patients that you have no magic, they think you the most powerful of all. Who but a real Merlin would deny power? Recall the temptations of Christ. This unrealistic—really irrational—approach is why it is said that the doctor who treats himself has a fool for a patient.

Childhood intrudes in other ways when we are sick. We want—we need—to be absolved of responsibility. We want—we need—to be taken care of. Emotional regression is a component of serious—particularly acute—illness. Even when not acutely ill we want the doctor to love us, to care. We resent paternalism but one part of us demands it. People are complex. The departing patient, at the end of a visit, would often ask, "When do you want to see me again?" "When you need me," I would reply, for I feel the role of a good doctor is to keep the patient well and out of the office. But that reply had the danger of being construed as not caring. "You don't love me," some buried part of the patient might think, never reflecting the job of the doctor (the real love) is to keep the patient independent. Thus the paradox. We want patient participation in decisions about treatment but the patient is the least well-poised individual to decide. And there is no one else to whom to turn.

A colleague of mine, an oncologist who had known me for years, knew my conservative outlook, knew my style of dealing with patients, came to see me many years ago having had his first nocturnal seizure. An adult life first nocturnal seizure often signals a temporal lobe tumor. Computerized tomography was still in its infancy so a first generation scan was unrevealing. Part of this may have been due to the technical quality of the first generation CT scan, but a working dictum even with later generation scanners was that the combination of a first adult life seizure and a negative CT scan implied a primary brain tumor; because the tumor is made up of brain tissue it may not be distinguishable from adjacent normal brain during its early stages of development. I suspected a brain tumor, elected to treat the seizure with medication, said nothing about my presumption (after all, I did not have a confirmed diagnosis—let the burden be mine rather than my patient's until I was certain) and arranged for a semiannual CT scan. Subsequent scans remained unrevealing of a tumor for about two and one half years during which my colleague, free of seizures, continued his practice, enjoyed family life and watched his children grow up. Then the tumor appeared on CT. "What do we do?" he asked. I suggested we continue what we had been doing. I explained what he, as an oncologist already knew. Treatment of brain tumors was unsatisfactory. Chemotherapy and radiation might add about six months to life at the end while taking time and quality of life at the beginning. It seemed to me best to make the most of the good time. My patient understood, he was educated in this field. But he needed action, he needed magic. Do something, do anything, but at least do *something*. He stayed with me for about two months, then I had a call from another neurologist at another hospital. "Dr. Oncol has come to me for treatment of his brain tumor. Now you know that I agree with you that aggressive treatment is futile but we both know that if I do not treat him he will continue to look around until he finds someone who will. So, if it's OK with you I'll arrange for x-ray therapy at my hospital." I said "Of course" and that I understood. My patient gave up his practice, lost his hair, grew a beard, had the sense that something was being done and that the magic might work. He died a short time later and autopsy showed the tumor had been unresponsive to therapy.

A doctor cannot impose his treatment decisions lest he be thought paternalistic. The best that can be suggested is to choose your doctor carefully and then follow his or her advice. However, for many patients it is not possible to choose a doctor; the insurance program makes you take what you get. And what you get may not be the same from day to day. There may be no real continuity of care. Take Intensive Care Units as an example.

A given doctor may be on duty for a specified period to be succeeded by a colleague. The baton is passed but the second member of the relay is never as fully informed as the first participant. Or the second doctor may have different methods of handling a given clinical situation. Continuity of care relies on the youngest member of the group—the resident—who remains present as the attendings rotate. And it relies on the computer where all the decisions and changes of decisions are recorded.

The computer offers one of the greatest changes in the practice of medicine, and one of the greatest temptations to cheat. The purpose of having three separate young doctors—a student, an intern, and a resident—take a history from and examine a hospital patient is to obtain three separate evaluations. Often it is the student's history that is most extensive, most complete, and most helpful. Today's House Staff cannot resist the temptation to download the history (and even the examination) of the first one to see the patient, and incorporate it into what is supposed to be an original document. After all, it saves time; you might even say it is efficient. It deprives the patient of a proper assessment and the young doctor of a chance to learn. But it is efficient.

Another way the computer has debased hospital care relates to nursing notes. At one time, they were a secret source of incisive information about the patient. Many doctors did not read them; I found the handwritten nurses notes to contain some of the most useful information sometimes unwittingly provided. Then came the time saving computer, which offers a list for the nurse to check off in each of a number of categories. Much faster, more efficient but if an item of importance is not on the checklist it does not get recorded. What may have been an essential nursing observation is overlooked. It is true the nurse can always add a handwritten note to the checklist but the very nature of checking things off tends to preclude any supplement.

Many things one would never consider are of importance to the hospitalized patient. One elderly, distinguished lady pointed out that lying in bed a prominent aspect of the doctor standing at the bedside (if he is a man) is his tie. The doctor's tie set a tone, conveyed a message of optimism or of uncertainty. Who would ever have guessed that? (Do doctors still wear ties?) Another elderly, dignified lady was outraged that on rounds the morning after abdominal surgery, her surgeon asked "How do you feel today Jean?" "Does he think" she asked, "that just because he looked at the inside of my belly he's entitled to call me by my first name?" (Do doctors—or anyone else—still use last names and the words Mr. or Mrs.?)

Yet another patient—a psychiatrist—was troubled that his surgeon never sat down during a visit. "Even if he stayed for only two minutes" said the psychiatrist "sitting down carries a different message than standing above the patient". These unintended messages, though unintended, may actually represent something of which the doctor is unaware, and of which the doctor should be aware.

Then there was the crusty old man I was asked to see in the hospital. "Who're you?" he demanded before I had a chance to introduce myself. I told him my name and explained that I was a consultant in neurology who had been asked by his doctor to examine him. "I'll tell you something," he said. "There was this fella had a Tom cat that used to go out on the Town every night and raise such a howl that the neighbors complained. So his owner took him to the vet and had him fixed. He still goes out on the Town every night, but now he's a consultant." How to maintain one's dignity and go on with the business at hand? It turned out that like every cranky old man he was really a softie underneath and grateful for my participation.

Everything about the patient and family can be used for diagnosis. I had a call from a woman requesting an appointment because she had a vaginal discharge. Was she telling me something? I explained I was a neurologist. "Oh", she said, "I got mixed up. My doctor gave me two names. One for my vaginal discharge and one for my son Donald's headaches." Confusion? Dementia? Or simply, she came first. "How old is Donald?" I asked, for I did not see pediatric patients. "He's eighteen," she said. The obvious question is why didn't Donald make his own appointment? When the time came, I greeted Donald in the waiting room. His mother—a large woman—marched into the office first and headed straight for my chair—an overstuffed easy chair in front of the desk, but facing into the room so there would be no barrier between doctor and patient, and so that I could see patients legs as well as their hands in their laps. It was obviously the doctor's chair—the chair of the person in charge. We got this straightened out. I heard the story of Donald's headaches and sent him into the examining room to get ready. While he was undressing, his mother said, "You might think I'm a possessive, overbearing mother and that I'm the cause of Donald's headaches; but look at it from my point of view. I'm 52, my husband is dead, my son is all I've got." Donald was my patient, so I was *his* advocate, but she was also right. You may remember the old story of the feudal lord called upon to adjudicate a dispute between two of his serfs. He heard the plaintiff and said, "You're right". He then listened to the defendant and said, "You're right". A friend said to him, "You can't do that. You can't say the plaintiff is right and then say the defendant is right" The lord turned to him and said, You're right too." I heard nothing from Donald or his mother for ten years. Presumably, my suggestions had been helpful. Then one day Donald, certain I did not remember him, phoned to say he needed to see me. When he arrived, he explained his headaches were OK, but he needed advice. He was still working as a master mechanic at the same luxury auto dealership, living with a girlfriend (I picture her as a blond) four or five days a week and with another girl friend (I think of her as a brunette) on weekends. He was now 28, he said, and thought it was time to get married, but could not decide which girl to choose. Could I help him? He still needed a mother, and would, I suppose, for his entire life.

What happens when the doctor becomes complicit in the financial aspects of patient care? This can occur in as least two ways. Physician members of an HMO may be penalized financially if they order what the HMO administration judges to be an excessive number of laboratory tests or use an excessive number of referrals. This is true whether physician compensation is based on capitation or not. Capitation consists of prospective payment of a fixed amount for each patient in the practice with bonuses or debits a result of tests and treatments. Alternatively, small groups of doctors—so called PODS—may share in the insurance savings or the deficits they have engendered which may range on the downside from as little as 10% to a full 100% depending on the contract negotiated. Suddenly financial considerations may contaminate medical judgement. What a given patient needs may be determined in part by what will provide the greatest financial return. Diagnostic testing may be reduced, out of network referrals eliminated, cheaper drugs chosen over better ones. Because, depending on the contract, the doctors may be financially responsible for the monetary loss caused the insurer by the care of their patients. Therefore, a POD—a group of physicians—may be liable for $100,000 (a not impossible figure) for a given financial quarter. A POD of ten physicians, faced with a potential debt of $40,000 each at the end of the year are also faced with a powerful incentive to cut back on patient "care". The criterion of good care shifts from what is best for the patient to what is best for the doctor, and ultimately what is best for the insurance carrier.

Physician tiering is a relatively new scheme to "improve health care quality while reducing costs". (For Your Benefit, Fall 2008) It is part of a "Pay for Performance" employed by more than 100 Health Plans. Physicians are divided into three tiers determined by quality and cost efficiency. Outpatient copays are determined by the level of the physician. In Minnesota members of the Advantage Health Plan who have completed a health risk assessment during the open enrollment period copay $17 at level 1, $22 for level 2, $27 for level 3 and $37 for level 4 physicians. Members who have not completed the health risk assessment are charged higher copays. A similar program is in effect for in hospital copays, and also for direct hospital reimbursement from Medicare, with up to 2% bonus in addition to standard payment. Programs of this sort put the diagnostic and therapeutic aspects of patient care on a financial basis. The worse the disease, the less good the outcome, and the less the financial incentive to care for seriously ill patients.

The Pay for Performance program—difficult to implement with individual practitioners—pays for treatment not for patient care. A number of criteria are evaluated and rewarded in the case of specific illnesses. Acute heart attack is one and such things as aspirin on arrival and aspirin on discharge are assessed. The Pay for Performance insurance program does not pay for activities that do not involve direct (that is, face to face) contact with the patient. Telephone calls (to patients, to other physicians or to insurer) are not reimbursed. Thinking is less rewarded than doing; cognitive activities gain less reimbursement than procedures. " . . . modifying *consumer* and *provider behavior* is one of the keys to increasing the level of quality and reducing the rising cost of health care" points out a brochure (The Clinical Performance Improvement Initiative and Physician Tiering) distributed by Unicare State Indemnity Plan which does not cover anesthesiologists, radiologists, hospitalists, pathologists, emergency room physicians, intensivists or psychiatrists. Quality is measured by the number and types of tests and procedures employed in a given clinical condition as compared with an "expected" quality compliance rate determined by a comparison with a group of peers. Cost efficiency is measured separately by comparing resource use of a physician with a group of peers. Although alleged to measure two separate factors to determine physician tier, it seems to me that ultimately both measures are of financial expenditure rather than quality of care, and neither deals with care, but instead with treatment. And so, the brochure advises the patient to become a "prudent buyer". This conflation of "quality" and "cost" makes it unlikely the suggestion of professional organizations to "ensure that rankings for doctors is not based solely on cost of care" and that "cost ratings alone should not be used to select physicians" (American Academy of Neurology Professional Association Position of the Principles of Physician Profiling" as an example) will be realized. The tiering program has generated considerable controversy and even litigation. In August 2008 the Massachusetts Medical Society announced it had filed legal action to correct the wrongs of the physician-ranking program. The major problem claimed is the ranking of physicians "using inaccurate, unreliable, and invalid tools and data" They write, "Doctors have been rated on procedures they have never done. They have been rated on patients they have never seen. The same doctor may be rated different ways by different health plans." One physician found her ranking adversely affected by her willingness to treat seriously ill patients who required resource intensive and multidisciplinary treatment. Another physician, on reviewing his assessment, found he was evaluated for patients he had never seen; he had only read their electrocardiograms. Similar suits have been filed by medical societies in Connecticut and Washington State.

The financial incentive for physicians—up to 10% of their reimbursement—depending on individual scores discourages taking care of severely or chronically ill patients. Part of the problem relates to the difficulty of establishing measurement criteria particularly for specialists. One of the larger participating physician networks has 3500 specialists. A unified measurement system has not been provided. Different insurers that use a Pay for Performance program use different measurement criteria, and outcome of treatment, which is perhaps the most objective criterion, is also one of the least suitable, excluding from compassionate treatment those who need it most. Still, a Press Release from the Center for Medicare and Medicaid Services of the Department of Health and Human Services in January 2005, discussing Medicare Pay for Performance initiatives says it "rewards physicians for improving health care outcomes". Clearly, the determinant of level of assignment is financial—i.e. cost savings. One insurance plan indicates, "Quality of care measurement is based on each physician's overall compliance rate against a set of clinical guidelines for recommended care". That must mean recommended care is determined by financial criteria. Non-financial incentives for physicians are also used, the most common of which is public reporting of performance. All of this variation, dissatisfaction, confusion, and turmoil may increase the pressure for a single payer system or at least a single set of mandated guidelines. A recent advertisement by Physicians for a National Health Program, advocated by more than 5000 physicians, indicates a potential annual savings of greater than 300 billion dollars "enough to cover the uninsured and to eliminate co-payments and deductibles for all Americans" (New Yorker Magazine October 13, 2008).

For physicians the lack of uniformity in guidelines creates a time consuming, non-medical involvement with the patient, or more accurately with the patient's insurance coverage, but the time consumed must be taken from time that should be devoted to a patient's medical needs. Using Medicare as an example of the five types of Advantage Plans compatible with Medicare coverage (Preferred Provider Organization, Health Maintenance Organization, Private Fee for Service Plan, Medical Savings Account, and Special Needs Plan) in two, the patient needs to choose a primary care physician, in the other three, not. Four allow care from any doctor (sometimes at a higher cost) the fifth requires the use of a network doctor. Two require referral to a specialist, three do not. Three cover prescribed drugs, one does not, and the fifth does sometimes. A given patient will know what the coverage allows; a given doctor—who is also concerned about tests, procedures, and referrals—will not, without investment of time. How much simpler it would be were there a universal standard or set of guidelines the insurance industry elected to embrace. Original Medicare could serve as an example for such things as tests (x-rays, EKG, MRI, CT), screenings (mammograms, prostate, pap tests, colonoscopy, bone density) as well as medically necessary services and hospital admissions. Catastrophic coverage, as part of, or in addition to each insurance plan should be mandatory so, for example, the young family, never anticipating the statistically unlikely event, will be protected. Most important the criteria should clearly enunciate whether they are aimed at the treatment of disease or care of a sick patient and disambiguate the two, so that a patient can understand in advance just what the insurance coverage offers.

WHITHER HENCE

Where to go from here? It is clear there is no going back. The days of caring for the patient are outdated; there are cynics who would argue that we cared for patients because we could not treat them. That is all we could do—offer compassion. So perhaps the first thing to do is draw a clear distinction between the care of the patient and the treatment of disease, and decide which is the role of the doctor, recognizing that it need not be one or the other. But if it is to be both, it will be more expensive than dealing with only one, and that one must be the treatment of disease, which is why "standard of care", a term employed by the insurance carriers, is not standard of care; it is standard of treatment. However, compassionate care alone is not enough, except perhaps in the case of an incurable disorder in its terminal phase.

This brings up the whole question of values. Not only health values but societal values in general, for health values, and the changes in the past decades, are a reflection of societal values and the changes in them. Social responsibility has yielded to personal aggrandizement. Money has become the yardstick of success. Good behavior and duty are unfamiliar concepts. And this change has been paralleled—actually resulted—in the changes in the practice of medicine and attitudes toward health. Is health important? Is health care important? Are they the same thing? How much are they worth? What percent of GDP? How many multimillion-dollar movies? Health care, which is so expensive, is provided after the effect of tobacco, of obesity or any other of the many preventables has done its mischief. Everyone agrees prevention is cheaper than treatment, but prevention infringes on personal and commercial interests. In addition, commercial interests fight a stubborn battle. Slowly the role of tobacco as a source of ill health is yielding to public pressure, but the battle persists. Perhaps the battlefield should be moved from the producer to the consumer. Excessive cigarette taxes might be more effective in discouraging smoking than all the advertising threats of cancer or other disease, and more effective than reduced life insurance premiums. Health insurance premiums could legitimately be tied to tobacco use or to obesity without raising the moral problems of DNA testing or of family history. This simply moves the issue of preexisting disease to an earlier stage, a stage of increased liability created by behavior that is under voluntary control, unlike a genetic endowment or family history. Any adjustment of insurance premiums or benefits will affect subscriber, provider, or taxpayer. Perhaps it is most fair to put the burden on the individual subscriber based on chosen health (and therefore healthcare) risks such as tobacco. This, of course, still leaves the problem of the 47 million uninsured who could not pay a surcharge even if covered by a mandated government carrier.

However, all this deals with treatment of disease and treatment of disease will continue to improve with the continued scientific explorations taking place in the laboratory and in the clinic. The question is whether anything can be done to improve the care of the patient which means the behavior of the doctor and therefore of the hospital. Here the outlook is discouraging. The changed attitude in the practice of medicine simply reflects the changed attitude in all our social institutions, in society at large. "Ask not what your country can do for you" is a thing of the past. One senses a yearning, particularly among the young, for a less selfish society, but the young will quickly outgrow it. Narcissism, greed, suspicion, and hostility are prominent; compassion and kindness are looked on as obscuring an ulterior motive. If these attitudes are engrained by time students enter medical school there is no way a four-year formal education will reverse them. If the determinant of choice of career is income opportunity, then the wrong motivation brings students into the profession and is irreversible. As I drove my VW Beetle past the front of the hospital, I saw one of my trainees hurrying along. I asked if I could give him a lift. As he got in, he explained he was on his way to pick up his car that was being serviced at the Mercedes dealer so that he could get to his stockbrokers office before it closed. Can I teach that boy compassion?

Patient expectations will have to change, as has already started. Only the old timers (doctors and patients) who remember the old days still expect a personal relationship. Younger patients are prepared to accept an "off the rack" approach. It does not matter who the doctor is; it does not matter whether the doctor is personally involved. All that matters (unless you are too sick to care) is that you get the correct medicine and that your insurance covers your bill. The doctor can take a place alongside other craftsmen. But unlike other craftsmen the doctor cannot offer a tangible product. A cure is not a commodity and may or may not be the outcome no matter how skilled an artisan the doctor may be. A failed treatment, a poor outcome on the background of an impersonal relation is rather different from buying an automobile that turns out to be a lemon. Does it mean the doctor didn't care? Would this doctor do better with involvement that is more personal? Could another doctor have done better? Should I sue? Malpractice suits can often be avoided by signs to the family that the doctor cares about a bad outcome, that the loss of a patient is painful. But that cannot be faked; the doctor must really care.

It is too late. Money has become the driving force for hospital and doctor, and that force cannot be reversed unless the current financial crisis so destroys economic society that it is ready for a new (or return to the old "brother's keeper") morality. And with it a sense of art, of how a thing is fashioned. I have cured some patients but had the sense it was done poorly, it had no style, it lacked grace. And I have lost some patients; they died but left me with a sense of a job well done. I had helped them and the departure had been graceful for patient and for family. I never liked to lose a patient but to fight a pointless battle insistently (and ruthlessly) with the aid of bottles and tubes is to inflict a sense of arrogance on a helpless patient and on a distraught family. The practice of medicine was an art—a long art that took years of experience and maturity to acquire—and still should be so; different from the science of treating disease.

If that art were to be retrieved—an impossible venture—it would require a reconstruction of the whole system. It would start, in my judgement, with a liberal education in college based on the classics and history, to develop a sense of human values. The required science courses would be in addition to rather than in exchange for. At the college level, the decision should be made as to whether the student is to become a treating, compassionate, bedside physician or a research scientist. Both, under this proposal, could obtain the MD degree, but the bifurcation into an ultimate clinical or research track should be clear from the start. The research candidate could have greater exposure to advanced college science courses, the ultimate clinician greater immersion in philosophy, ethics, and the humanities. This is not a generally accepted approach. A recent report on restructuring premedical education (New England Journal of Medicine July 17, 2008) continues to emphasize the sciences and biological relevance giving only token acknowledgement to ethics, altruism, and compassion, which are "best reserved for medical schools". Graduates of the two tracks of college premedical programs should both go to medical school, both should do internships, both should obtain state licenses (in order to have access to patients) but only one should do research (clinical or laboratory) and only the other should care for patients. This will abolish the current "on service" problem—the problem of not being able to obtain a desired hospital consultant because this is a research, not a clinical, month. However, it will also necessitate a restructuring of medical school appointments, giving clinical faculty the same opportunities and prestige as research faculty. Promotion should not be based solely on publication or investigative achievement. This is not to suggest that research could no longer take place in the hospitals or that clinical faculty could not collaborate. It is simply to remove research interests from intruding on the primary concern of patient care. Medical schools could continue the trend to move patient contact into earlier years, and increased primary care or family medicine should be made available for those on the clinical track, for this exposure will increase awareness of human aspects of the practice of medicine. At the same time, the research track student could have access to an MDPhD program of the sort now available at many medical schools.

Postgraduate teaching in the hospital needs a major revision. (Keep in mind that what I am proposing is fantasy; it will not occur, though it should). Large cadres of residents, remote professors concerned only with the academic aspects of training, do not work. Resident programs must be small, even for the intellectual, academic aspects. At a time when our training program involved three hospitals through which the House Officers rotated, when corrected about some point or other a typical reply by the resident would be "That's not how they do it across the street" no matter how they did it across the street. In any case, that reply was arrogant backtalk and an impediment to learning. Even if the correction were to be rejected, the trainee would do well to listen silently, consider, then reject rather than engage contentiously. But self-esteem requires expression of one's self assurance. If it is argued that hospitals cannot reduce the size of the resident staff, at least the resident staff can be divided into small cohorts (let's say no more than five individuals) responsible to a single staff instructor who supervises only one group continuously for the entire academic year. And like a squad or small platoon, overseen by a staff sergeant, the staff member must exert extreme discipline by example and by demands. Insubordination must not be tolerated, group pride and morale must devolve, peer pressure must develop, and a tradition of patient care must be instituted. It should be considered a privilege to be a team member and privilege brings responsibility. Good behavior should be rewarded, bad behavior punished. The rewards and punishment can be the tokens of group approval or rejection. Attitudes and behaviors begin with the staff member and are passed down the line to the newest recruit. To remain in good standing in this prestigious group one must accept responsibility, pull one's own weight. For House Staff to know their patients (without notes) and to take their responsibility as a moral commitment, the caseload must be manageable. This may entail a large number of teams with the associated economic problems of more residents and staff members to be paid. Federal funds will continue under existing Direct and Indirect Graduate Medical Education programs, which provide payments to hospitals for the costs of approved graduate medical education. These programs reflect the higher patient care costs of teaching hospitals compared with non teaching hospitals and are based on hospital

Medicare payments. Sources of supplementary income are limited: 1—the hospital staff—professional and administrative 2—the patient 3—the government. 1—Can staff be tithed? Is it appropriate that some physicians and hospital administrators make in excess of one million dollars a year? Should they contribute to the education and support of the resident staff, which, in turn, is helping them? A physician's job would be much harder without the presence of the "on call" resident. Should there be a cap on physician remuneration, with excess income generated applied to resident training? One way, but a bad way, to do this is by tying annual salary to academic level. Another way would be years of service, with reimbursement consisting of a combination of hospital salary related to teaching and supervision supplemented by clinical, patient generated income. Should patient generated income exceed the cap, a small amount—say 25%—could be returned to the physician and the remainder applied to expenses resulting from the resident platoon system. 2—Should the patient assume part of the financial burden of resident training? After all, the patient is the recipient of the 24 hour on duty program provided by the House Staff. In a sense, this is nothing more than an extension of the concierge system to the hospital. A patient or family could elect to join for the duration of the hospital stay and a predetermined surcharge could be applied to the hospital bill (either a percentage or more equitably, a fixed daily fee) in exchange for which the patient has an assigned resident. Those who do not join are not assigned House Staff. However, like the "scholarship patients" of a concierge program, one House Staff platoon on a rotating basis would assume emergency responsibility for unassigned patients

3-Should the Federal government provide additional training grants independent of Medicare provisions (as it has done in previous years) to assist in the postgraduate training of young doctors? This would provide on the clinical side the counterpart of research grants on the laboratory side. Government funds should most reasonably be provided in a lump sum—determined by the number of trainees—(to the hospital, or less effectively to the medical school for redistribution to the hospital) in response to an annual application specifying needs and methods of use. These funds, if awarded, would be used to supplement, not replace, current existing sources of resident support. Alternatively, the individual resident could apply directly (to the hospital or even to the Government program) for supplementary funds. Recommendations by staff would serve as criteria, and would function as financial incentive to the resident for responsible, concerned behavior.

The major change in the resident training program must be in the discipline of the young trainee. At the outset of the academic year, an inflexible set of rules and expectations must be provided. These should have been made available to applicants to the training program so they knew in advance what to expect, and had opportunity to decline applying. The rules should specify responsibilities and obligations, and indicate a chain of command and an appeal process. As a working rule, the chain of command should support the decision of the next lower member as long as such support is equitable. The Chief of Service must support his faculty even though concerned with getting sufficient House Staff applicants. Otherwise, discipline breaks down. The manipulative intern plays one staff member against another as a manipulative child pits father against mother. Individual House Staff must not be allowed to change the rules capriciously and at will to suit individual needs. Rules represent departmental policy, must be enforced impartially, and must serve as criteria for reappointment. Reappointment should be annual for House Staff (at many hospitals it is every two years for regular staff, with reapplication and review by the Credentials Committee required) with criteria specified at the time of initial application into the program, so unsatisfactory performance by unwilling participants can result in failure of reappointment. A decision to terminate a trainee's appointment at the end of an academic year is not considered a disciplinary action if done for reasons other than conduct or performance, is not entitled to appeal and is therefore without the option of litigation. In Massachusetts, disciplinary action must be reported to the Board of Registration in Medicine.

The written rules and expectations should be provided to each faculty member so there be no misunderstandings, for faculty are the enforcers. Misunderstandings occur when the faculty are not clear about or have unrealistic expectations just as when the trainee does not understand or chooses to ignore what is expected. Expectations are codified by the Accreditation Council of Graduate Medical Education, which oversees and certifies group performance just as the professional Boards certify individual performance. ACGME lists as one of its requirements (July 1, 2007) "Residents must demonstrate a commitment to carrying out professional responsibilities and an adherence to ethical principles. Residents are expected to demonstrate: 1—compassion, integrity and respect for others; 2—responsiveness to patient needs that supersedes self-interest; 3—respect for patient privacy and autonomy; 4—accountability to patients, society, and the profession;" If ACGME guidelines are not followed—a responsibility of the faculty, not the trainee—accreditation of the program may be withdrawn. Much of the ACGME concern is to support the trainee, so discipline for behavior becomes difficult; and how to instill compassion, integrity, respect, accountability, and lack of self-interest is not specified. The treatment of disease and the correction of treatment mistakes are easy to teach and to discipline. Responsibility, behavior and style are harder to teach (the ethicist might even argue we have no right to try, no authority to control or shape another's personality) but these are the very factors that make a good doctor. How quickly to respond to a patient's needs, how involved to become, how personally concerned. The quantifiable aspects of style (such as how soon after admission a hospitalized patient must be seen, or how quickly an admission note must be available) can be specified in the statement of expectations; the rest must be learned (if it is to be learned at all) by the examples set by the faculty members in their own performance.

Just as I believe resident programs profit from a reduction in size and a greater sense of cohesion, so, I believe, the staff pyramid should be reshaped. With ten professors, for example, in a department that previously had one, it is now top heavy, particularly from an administrative viewpoint. The first question to be addressed is whether the elevation to a professorship is a sign of true academic achievement or is simply an expression of loyalty, friendship, or financial endowment generated. If, as I propose, there is a division of staff into clinical and research faculties the question of professorship becomes complicated; professorships usually indicate scholarly achievement. Clinical activities—particularly teaching—are essential in a training environment but do not produce tangible scholarly results of the sort that usually constitute criteria for appointment to a professorship. One way to deal with this is to restore the old classification of Clinical Professor but that was always considered a somewhat inferior appointment—not the "real thing". A better way, in my judgement, is to limit the number of professors in a department to one, in charge of clinical and research functions as well as administrative aspects of the department. At the next lower level—call it associate professor—come the senior clinical and research members of the department, in charge of teaching and laboratories. Their status and salaries are comparable one with the other, and no prestige distinction is made between clinical and research appointments. Just as the clinical staff can generate bonuses from clinical activity, so research faculty can supplement their incomes from research grants, honoraria and consulting fees, with a cap similar to that of clinical practice of 25% above base negotiated salary. If tithing is an acceptable approach, the tithe could be provided from the excess funds generated above the 25% bonus to the clinical or research individual.

From the patient's point of view the best thing that could happen would be to return to the fee for service system and free choice of physician. This would restore to the patient the power that was ceded to the insurance industry. The patient could negotiate directly with the physician whose responsibility would now be exclusively to the patient. Patient satisfaction would once again become important because if unsatisfied the patient could seek care elsewhere. However, unlike the old fee for service system, an insurance program similar to the original Medicare could now undertake this. It need not be a single payer system (although there is no reason why is should not be) but all companies should follow the same rules and same payment schedule if only to reduce physician confusion that exists under the current programs of differing rules and payments. Patients could select their physicians, not be restricted to a single primary care physician, and have unlimited access including specialists. Coverage should be universal. This could be a government program—federal or state—either in its entirety or as a supplement to private insurance so the government becomes the agent for the currently uninsured 47 million. Programs based on a Medicare template would have to duplicate part A and B coverage so that physicians as well as hospitals were paid. As with Medicare part B the physician should have the option of accepting assigned payment or not. If not, payment becomes the patient's responsibility; in return, the patient receives the assigned amount as reimbursement. If this is not satisfactory to the patient, care can be transferred to a doctor who accepts assignment. Medication must be covered, generic drugs must be mandated, physicians should be encouraged to use the cheapest satisfactory drugs (a recommended formulary could be provided) and money saving scams by the insurer should be outlawed. For example, at one time insulin for diabetics was covered by insurance but needles and syringes were not; how the diabetic patient was expected to administer the insulin was not indicated by this insurance program.

Of course, all of this is fantasy. It will not happen. Current attitudes and procedures will persist and progress inexorably. The patient will be dehumanized and concomitantly so will the doctor. The major complaint from still practicing old time physicians is some variation of "It's not fun anymore" or "I don't enjoy my work now". The thinking physician is no longer necessary; and thinking was fun. God is now in the machine. Technology makes the diagnosis; the physician becomes a technician. Not even that, for it is not necessary to run the machine or even to know how the machine is run. It is enough simply to order the test. Instead of being a tool to be used by the physician, the physician has become a tool to be used by the machine. We used to give postgraduate seminars to which physicians from all over the country would come. Some would bring tape recorders, which would be turned on, at the beginning of the lecture. Its owner would promptly fall asleep as the machine did the listening. Even there the machine had replaced the doctor. Most of the time the machine will be right, will make the correct diagnosis (if the right machine has been chosen). If it does not, nobody is to blame. No individual is at fault; a machine made a mistake. The medical student is no longer interested in learning physical diagnosis; the machine will do it (New England Journal of Medicine February 9, 2006).

Just as the physician is replaced by the machine, so, in a curious way, is the patient. Patients may no longer present unfiltered symptoms. Instead, they offer diagnoses and requests for remedies suggested by the internet, by television or by home remedy manuals. It becomes increasingly difficult to obtain raw data; "Tell me what you feel not what you think" is a vain request. A knowledgeable patient is a good thing because it helps a patient understand a doctor's reasoning, but the patient's knowledge should not replace the doctor. Patients have a remarkable way of being correct, of knowing what is wrong, but not when they try to usurp the role of doctor; only when, without effort, they allow intuition to work. I would often ask patients at the end of an examination "What do you think is wrong?" and on occasion would be rewarded with a correct diagnosis. There is an old study allegedly reporting visits to physicians by middle-aged men who did not usually go to doctors. Symptoms were vague, diagnoses often not made. Within the next several weeks' heart attacks occurred. These men knew something was wrong. Physicians must listen carefully in this kind of situation; patients must not try to diagnose. And machines will be of little help; they do not know the right questions to ask.

What will need to happen is for attitudes to change. Those of us who entered the profession with one set of attitudes and found ourselves practicing under another are gradually disappearing. Today's medical students presumably know what they will encounter and are prepared. Patient expectations must also change. Those who anticipate a personal relationship will be disappointed. They will gradually diminish in number as the reality of the medical world conditions patients to accommodate to what might be called veterinary medicine—the treatment of disease. And the treatment of disease, which is the important factor, will improve thanks largely to our research colleagues.

Perhaps the hospital Pastoral Services will replace the personal concern of the old time physician. However, pastoral participation is usually a part time adjunct to a congregation elsewhere. The pastoral departments are often understaffed, available on a rotating, so therefore an impersonal, basis, and when available are often rushed. Even under ideal circumstances, pastoral counseling is best used as a supplement to, rather than as a replacement of, medical counseling and care. And, of course, in hospital pastoral care will not be available on an outpatient (that is, office) basis. It is in the office where most medical care occurs and where the personal relation with the physician is needed to generate confidence, patient understanding, and compliance.

What about the three divisions of the medical community and the dynamic tension among them that maintains a balance of interest? A fourth force has been introduced to destabilize the balance—the insurance industry that consumes about 25% of the premiums that should be applied for health care. The influence of that industry—really the control it exerts—is on the doctors and hospitals it supports and not, as it should be, as the guardian of the sick patient. It has co-opted the hospitals and doctors by the financial return which has deputized (perhaps unwillingly in the case of the doctors) them. Hospitals still turn to their communities (usually former patients) in their financial appeals, but are fundamentally impelled by a profit motive. Insurance income, generated by procedures and services should cover expenses, so procedures and services are encouraged. Doctor's incomes, too, are tied to what is done, so doctors are tempted to do too much. The counterpoise is the effort by the insurance industry to reduce costs, reduce their financial outlay, and increase their profits. This can only be done by limiting procedures and services through a series of permissions and controls. The dynamic tension shifts to the doctors and hospitals on one side and the insurance industry on the other. The patient, who once played a role in the triumvirate, is now a passive bystander on the sidelines, to be manipulated by the participants. Even the participants are manipulated, for doctors and hospitals have little negotiating power. The insurers tell them what they will be paid, what they may do or not do, and the doctors may be financially penalized or rewarded for their behavior. Perhaps a capitation program helps with some aspects of the imbalance, but it brings with it other problems; it may reduce the tendency for excessive services but it also reduces the personal relationship between doctor and patient. So, it seems to me, the best compromise is a fee for service insurance program of the kind initiated by the original Medicare mandate.

"What's old collapses, times change," says Schiller (William Tell IV ii). And so it has been. Care of the patient is no longer a medical priority. Once I had thought the pendulum would swing back, but no longer. The concerned, sympathetic physician has been replaced by the impersonal, financially motivated technician. What can we salvage? The first thing should be the independence, the dignity, and the concerns of the patient. The power (to use a clumsy term) of the patient must be restored. That power, in the current health care marketplace is financial. Financial strength that can only be restored by giving the potential patient financial independence, which in turn, endows freedom, flexibility and a voice in the marketplace. This can be done without a major dislocation in the current financial organization of the insurance industry simply by establishing an open marketplace on the pattern of the original Medicare program. The patient has freedom of choice of physician and receives, as a result, a personal relationship. The physician is reimbursed at a reasonable rate (the Medicare rate could serve as a guide) and retains the ability to accept or refuse assigned payment. Physician judgement once again becomes the determinant of tests and procedures. Insurance company judgements become the determinant of whether or by how much tests and procedures are reimbursed. A physician who orders unnecessary tests or procedures will shortly enough face peer pressure (from unreimbursed colleagues) to desist or at least to change criteria. Insurance companies must exercise good judgement in disallowing payment and there must be an appeal mechanism with generous professional representation.

This still leaves the problem of the uninsured who crowd Emergency Rooms, where they receive more costly care than they would were they insured. What that seems to say is that everyone should be covered. The Massachusetts experiment may be the first step in that direction and could serve as a bellwether. Government coverage of the uninsured—whether federal on a Medicare model or state on a Massachusetts model—may turn out to be financially prudent as well as morally correct. It would restore patient dignity and physician commitment to provide care to all. Finally, one can only dream of a return of the concepts of responsibility, duty, morality and perhaps even good manners.

www.ingramcontent.com/pod-product-compliance
Lightning Source LLC
Chambersburg PA
CBHW022125170526
45157CB00004B/1751